ADVANCE

Plant-Powe

"In *Plant-Powered for Life*, Sharon Palme.   into an absolutely delightful culinary adventure. The fabulous recipes are inspired by traditions from around the world, and a clear understanding of food and health. This book is truly exceptional— from beginning to end, it is beautifully and brilliantly crafted." —BRENDA DAVIS, RD, coauthor of *Becoming Vegan*

"Nutrition science and sustainability are complex issues. Sharon has done a masterful job of simplifying the science with 52 recommendations that give the reader clear guidance on making choices that are good for personal health as well as the health of our planet. Her culinary talent shines through with 125 recipes inspired by plant-based cuisines and cultures from around the world. Reading this book will enhance your understanding of the science; cooking from this book will make shopping for, preparing, and cooking amazing meals satisfying and fun!"

—AMY MYRDAL MILLER, MS, RDN, Senior Director of Programs and Culinary Nutrition, The Culinary Institute of America

"Making healthy eating practical, realistic, and delicious—that's what Sharon Palmer is known for. Her tips for improving dietary choices are simple but powerful, and her recipes—inspired by the world's most appealing cuisines—will show you how to eat for good health while enjoying some of the best meals you've ever tasted." —VIRGINIA MESSINA, MPH, RD, coauthor of *Vegan for Life*, *Vegan for Her*, and *Never Too Late to Go Vegan*

"As you heed Sharon Palmer's advice to *fall in love with plants*, you will no doubt fall in love with Sharon's newest book. The pages of *Plant-Powered for Life* are filled with great tips and easy-to-follow, delicious-looking recipes that also happen to be incredibly healthy." —SARA BAER-SINNOTT, President, Oldways

"*Plant-Powered for Life* will give people a new appreciation for the dazzling and delicious variety plant foods offer. Sharon's 52 simple steps and 125 recipes will help eaters of all persuasions, from carnivores to vegans, make plant-based meals fun and exciting." —PEGGY NEU, President, The Monday Campaigns

"Sharon has done it again! Enjoy this brilliantly written book filled with easy-to-prepare recipes that are sure to delight the palate of those new to plant-based cuisine." —JOHN PIERRE, author of *The Pillars of Health: Your Foundations for Lifelong Wellness*, www.johnpierre.com

THE EXPERIMENT

BECAUSE EVERY BOOK IS A TEST OF NEW IDEAS

SELECTED PRAISE FOR

The Plant-Powered Diet

"Registered dietitian Sharon Palmer wrote a book that is much like a superfood: dense with the good stuff. The abundance of information in the first half is worth its weight in kale, then followed by 75 of the author's own, family-tested recipes. This is a tome ideal for flexitarians and new vegans who are still learning."

—VegNews.com

"In *The Plant-Powered Diet*, Sharon Palmer shares her passion for wholesome, delicious plant foods. This book, which is based on compelling scientific evidence, will help you find your own plant-based eating style that's healthy, sustainable, and delicious." —CHERYL FORBERG, RD, James Beard Award–winning chef, *New York Times* bestselling author, and original nutritionist for *The Biggest Loser*

"*The Plant-Powered Diet* makes the transition to a plant-powered lifestyle simple. The support tools, such as pantry lists, dining out tips, and recipes, will help anyone realistically make the leap into a plant-powered lifestyle. It's refreshing to see a focus on whole food, vegetarian recipes." —DAWN JACKSON BLATNER, RD, author of *The Flexitarian Diet*

"*A plant-powered diet* is a very powerful step in the right direction toward an all plant-based, whole-food diet. A very useful and very informative book."

—GENE STONE, editor of *Forks Over Knives: The Plant-Based Way to Health* and author of *The Secrets of People Who Never Get Sick*

"*The Plant-Powered Diet* is a compilation of compelling arguments for the ideal nutrition plan—one that is based on whole plant foods. Palmer is welcoming to her readers as she provides solutions for eating in a more health-promoting way. I recommend this as a resource for anyone seeking a healthier diet."

—JULIEANNA HEVER, MS, RD, CPT, plant-based dietitian and author of *The Complete Idiot's Guide to Plant-Based Nutrition*

"*The Plant Powered Diet* is a spot-on roadmap for our time. Eating deliciously, healthfully, and with a sense of our place in the world has never been easier, thanks to Sharon—I love this book!" —KATE GEAGAN, MS, RD, author of *Go Green Get Lean: Trim Your Waistline with the Ultimate Low-Carbon Footprint Diet*

"*The Plant-Powered Diet* is a celebration of the delicious, healthful qualities of beautiful plant foods in their natural form. Everyone can gain tremendous benefits from eating this way." —PATRICIA BANNAN, MS, RD, nutrition expert and author of *Eat Right When Time Is Tight*

PLANT-POWERED
FOR LIFE

Eat Your Way to Lasting Health

WITH 52 SIMPLE STEPS

& 125 DELICIOUS RECIPES

SHARON PALMER, RDN

Photography by Heather Poire

THE EXPERIMENT
NEW YORK

PLANT-POWERED FOR LIFE: *Eat Your Way to Lasting Health with 52 Simple Steps and 125 Delicious Recipes*

Copyright © 2014 Sharon Palmer
Photographs copyright © 2014 Heather Poire

All rights reserved. Except for brief passages quoted in newspaper, magazine, radio, television, or online reviews, no portion of this book may be reproduced, distributed, or transmitted in any form or by any means, electronic or mechanical, including photocopying, recording, or information storage or retrieval system, without the prior written permission of the publisher.

Many of the designations used by manufacturers and sellers to distinguish their products are claimed as trademarks. Where those designations appear in this book and The Experiment was aware of a trademark claim, the designations have been capitalized.

The Experiment, LLC
220 East 23rd Street, Suite 301
New York, NY 10010-4674
www.theexperimentpublishing.com

This book contains the opinions and ideas of its author. It is intended to provide helpful and informative material on the subjects addressed in the book. It is sold with the understanding that the author and publisher are not engaged in rendering medical, health, or any other kind of personal professional services in the book. The author and publisher specifically disclaim all responsibility for any liability, loss, or risk—personal or otherwise—that is incurred as a consequence, directly or indirectly, of the use and application of any of the contents of this book.

The Experiment's books are available at special discounts when purchased in bulk for premiums and sales promotions as well as for fund-raising or educational use. For details, contact us at info@theexperimentpublishing.com.

Library of Congress Cataloging-in-Publication Data

Palmer, Sharon.
  Plant-powered for life : eat your way to lasting health with 52 simple steps and 125 delicious recipes / Sharon Palmer, RDN.
     pages cm
  Includes index.
  ISBN 978-1-61519-187-1 (paperback) -- ISBN 978-1-61519-188-8 (ebook)
  1. Vegan cooking. 2. Cooking (Vegetables) 3. Cooking (Natural foods) 4. Vegan cooking--Health aspects.
  5. Natural foods. 6. Nutrition. I. Title.
   TX837.P26 2014
   641.5'636--dc23
                                        2013050760

ISBN 978-1-61519-187-1
Ebook ISBN 978-1-61519-188-8

Cover design by Laura Palese
Cover image © ithinksky | iStockPhoto
Author photograph © Vanessa Stump

Text design by Pauline Neuwirth, Neuwirth & Associates, Inc.

Manufactured in the United States of America
Distributed by Workman Publishing Company, Inc.
Distributed simultaneously in Canada by Thomas Allen & Son Ltd.

First printing May 2014
10 9 8 7 6 5 4 3 2 1

Contents

Introduction

If I were to offer one nugget of nutrition advice it would be to *fall in love with plants*. Because if you really, truly start loving plants—craving their flavors, textures, aromas, and colors—they will start loving you back. Whole plants, which have sustained humans throughout the centuries, possess the power to keep you healthy, functional, and fit—to help you live a long, rich, full life. It's that simple.

In the coming pages, I will illuminate this simple message and equip you with fifty-two equally simple habits that form the core of plant-powered eating, along with recipes to inspire and sustain you. One step at a time, I will take you on a journey toward optimal health and all the other delicious rewards that a diet rich in plants can provide. Along the way, you'll learn so many amazing things about plants that you'd need a heart of stone not to fall in love with them.

Every plant food—grain, legume, vegetable, fruit, nut, or seed—has a story to tell. Take the carrot, which began in Afghanistan as a purple or yellow root before Dutch growers took hold of a mutant orange carrot and developed the forefather of today's sweet, plump orange root. Or okra, which arrived in the United States via female slaves who tucked okra seeds—one of their most precious possessions—into their hair when they were stolen from their homes in West Africa.

Throughout history, people have collected and nurtured plants: plants were their sustenance, their medicine, their life. They traded their precious plants between their worlds—flax and dates from Mesopotamia, exotic spices from the East, and potatoes, tomatoes, and chocolate from the New World. Farmers began to save the seeds from their showiest, tastiest crops—from squash to corn—recognizing them as "heirlooms" to be treasured and planted the next year. And today, we have thousands of varieties of beautiful plants for the picking: take any vegetable—say, a tomato or bean—and you'll find that there are hundreds or sometimes thousands of different varieties. Even if you tried, it would be impossible to taste every type of edible plant available on the planet in one lifetime.

As humans were busy collecting, cultivating, and eating these precious plants, the plants were giving back. You might say the plants were "thanking" us for ensuring that their offspring survived for years to come. Their gift in return was good health. Each plant contained compounds that protected it from sun, insects, and disease, and bestowed vibrant health on its eater. The plants nourished our vision, our skin, our brains, and our hearts.

Today, by eating plants in their whole natural form—the way they grow in nature or on a farm—you can stoke your diet with all of the good stuff: fiber, protein, healthy fats, slow-burning carbs, vitamins, minerals, and phytochemicals (plant compounds with health-protective activity). Whether you are omnivorous, pescatarian, vegetarian, or vegan, you can gain benefits by making way for more whole plant foods.

As a registered dietitian and nutrition expert, I have helped thousands of people live healthier lives through diet. And as a journalist, I travel to nutrition conferences around the world, interview the leading nutrition researchers, and study published nutrition research every day in order to keep up on the body of evidence surrounding health and nutrition. This broad base of science points to one compelling fact: a whole-foods, plant-based diet is your best-odds defense against disease.

We must make a sure-footed move back toward the plants that sustained us. We must leave behind the typical American diet (or *Western diet*). This diet—laden with highly processed foods, fatty meats, saturated fat, sodium, and sugar, and pathetically deficient in whole plant foods like whole grains, legumes, vegetables, and fruits (and their star nutrients such as fiber, vitamins, and minerals)—is killing us. We struggle with a cascade of diet-related diseases: heart disease, obesity, type 2 diabetes, cancer, Alzheimer's disease, premature aging, early death, poor mental and physical functioning, and the list goes on.

Even our kids now face these diseases at an unprecedented rate. When I first started practicing as a dietitian, type 2 diabetes was called adult-onset diabetes, because it rarely occurred before the age of forty. Today, it happens in children, too. In addition, modern kids have strokes and are in the early stages of atherosclerosis (plaque buildup in the arteries), all as a result of their poor diets and lack of exercise. For the first time in history, our kids are set to live shorter lives than we will live.

As kids with early risk factors for diabetes and heart disease mature, our country will be saddled with poor health, medical bills, and disability. And the entire planet is already maxed out for resources: scientists say we would need one-and-a-half Earths to keep up with our consumption of food, water, and energy. You might be surprised to find that 51 percent of our greenhouse gas emissions are produced through resource-intensive animal agriculture. It's no longer sustainable to eat this way—for us, for our children, or for our planet.

Diet is a powerful ally that can literally save your life. You can reduce your risk of all these chronic diseases by 80 percent (yes, you read that right!) by embracing a healthy lifestyle that includes eating and drinking well, not smoking, and exercising. No drug on the market can boast those odds.

The optimal diet for a healthy life—and planet—is within our reach. It's so sweet and simple that it often goes unnoticed amid the thunder of fad diets. It's simply a diet that gets back to nature, to eating the simple whole foods that once nurtured us.

Since writing my first book, *The Plant-Powered Diet*, I've had the pleasure of hearing the success stories of so many people who made changes in their diet and reaped the rewards. Some people made huge changes by becoming vegan; other people made moderate changes, like cutting out red meat or eating a mostly plant-based diet. These changes resulted in wonderful success: weight loss; discontinuing medication for high blood pressure, diabetes, and high cholesterol; improvement in chronic disease symptoms; and beyond. Best of all, people have told me they just "feel good," in terms of both their health and their place in our food system. They are remarkably energized and involved in their relationship with food. They don't feel deprived or as if they were on a "diet"; instead they celebrate delicious, wholesome plant foods.

In the chapters of this new book, I hope that I inspire *you* to fall under the lure of plants—to savor and respect their nourishment, good taste, and gift of health. Start by setting a plant-powered goal of your own (see page 1), then proceed toward it step by step. You can tackle the steps in the order they're given, or skip around and choose your own pathway. Do one a week for a year, or take it at your own pace.

I also share 100 percent plant-based recipes to try in your kitchen. Drawing on the world's abundance of plant-powered ingredients and flavors, these dishes will reward your efforts with vibrant health *and* vibrant meals.

Each recipe is packed with the power of essential nutrients; when a recipe provides a good source (at least 10% Daily Value [DV], the requirement for the average adult, based on a 2,000-calorie diet) of a vitamin or mineral, it is listed as a "star nutrient." While I believe good nutrition is about *food* more than nutrients, I share this information to illustrate how plant foods can provide good sources of nutrients, like calcium, iron, and zinc. The nutrition information also includes calorie, protein, carbohydrate, fat, saturated fat, fiber, sugar (an amount that includes both added sugars and sugars that naturally occur in plant foods), and sodium content for each recipe, to help you make decisions based on your personal nutrition needs.

Every recipe also either is gluten-free or offers simple gluten-free substitutions. Certain ingredients (included but not limited to grains, flours, baking powder, and condiments, such as soy sauce) may contain gluten or be subject to cross-contamination, depending on the manufacturer. If you follow a gluten-free diet, read labels carefully and choose reliably gluten-free brands. Note that not everyone needs to follow a gluten-free diet: it can be as healthy as any other eating style, but is not necessarily better for you if you do not have celiac disease or another gluten-related disorder.

By taking each of this book's fifty-two steps and reinforcing them over time with your actions and your cooking, you'll steadily build new habits that will promote health throughout the year and across a lifetime. You'll also learn just how simple and delicious plant-based eating can be.

Your plant-powered life begins today—and once you've tasted the benefits, you'll never want it to end.

PLANT-
POWERED
FOR LIFE

Shanghai Stir-Fry
with Forbidden Rice

Create your own plant-powered goal.

Shanghai Stir-Fry with Forbidden Rice
Fettuccine with Romesco Sauce

No two people eat precisely alike. Some of us dine out twice a day; some of us rarely visit restaurants. Some of us eat meat every day; some of us never do. But we can all achieve sustainable health and well-being by focusing more on whole plant foods, and less on animal foods.

The first step is to create a personal goal on the plant-powered spectrum. You won't be "going on a diet," but committing to make concrete, lasting changes that work for you. If your goal changes over time, that's fine.

PLANT-POWERED VEGAN	PLANT-POWERED VEGETARIAN	PLANT-POWERED OMNIVORE
Excludes all animal foods, including dairy and eggs	Excludes all animal flesh, but includes dairy and eggs	Pescatarian: Excludes all animal flesh, except for seafood Semi-vegetarian: Eats a small amount of animal flesh

Take a look at how you eat every day, and ask yourself:

- How many servings of animal foods do you eat every day?
- How many servings of whole plant foods do you eat every day?
- When in the day do you tend to eat these foods?
- Which eating behaviors do you most want to change? (Perhaps you plan to give up processed meats, like bacon, sausage, and ham, which have been linked to an even higher risk of cancer, heart disease, and type 2 diabetes than other animal foods.)

Next, set your own plant-powered goal. Say it out loud! For example, depending on your personal goals, it might go something like:

- I will cut out red meat and eat a whole-foods, meatless meal once a week.
- I will eat dairy, eggs, fish, and whole plant foods.
- I will eat an entirely vegan plant-powered diet.

Now that you've set a goal, use this book to achieve it!

shanghai stir-fry with forbidden rice

One of the best ways to move to a plant-powered diet is to focus on dishes that showcase vegetables, such as this stir-fry, which includes a mix of traditional Chinese plant foods—bamboo shoots, water chestnuts, baby corn, carrots, Chinese cabbage, and bean sprouts. Add tofu, tempeh, or seitan for a punch of plant protein; omnivores may opt to stir in a small amount of lean meat or seafood as "seasoning." Loaded with flavor and texture, the colors of this stir-fry really pop when juxtaposed with jet-black "forbidden" rice—so precious that it was reserved for Chinese emperors.

MAKES 8 SERVINGS
(about 1¼ cups stir-fry with ½ cup rice each)

1⅓ cups (240 g) uncooked forbidden (black) rice
2⅓ cups (552 ml) water
1 tablespoon sesame oil
1 medium carrot, sliced (see Note)
1 medium onion, coarsely sliced
3 medium garlic cloves, minced
1½ teaspoons minced fresh ginger
1 tablespoon black sesame seeds
1 medium green bell pepper, coarsely sliced
One 15-ounce (425 g) can baby corn, drained (1¾ cups)
One 8-ounce (227 g) can water chestnuts, drained
One 8-ounce (227 g) can bamboo shoots, drained
3 cups (210 g) sliced Chinese (Napa) cabbage
1 cup (70 g) sliced mushrooms
1 cup (104 g) fresh bean sprouts
¼ cup (4 g) chopped fresh cilantro
3 tablespoons reduced sodium soy sauce
½ teaspoon rice vinegar
1 tablespoon agave nectar
¼ cup (59 ml) reduced sodium vegetable broth (see page 346)
1 tablespoon cornstarch
2 green onions, white and green parts, sliced
½ cup (69 g) coarsely chopped cashews

1. Place the rice and water in a small pot, cover, and simmer over medium-low heat for about 30 minutes, until tender, with all of the water absorbed.

2. Meanwhile, heat the sesame oil in a large sauté pan or wok over medium heat.

3. Add the carrot and onion and sauté for 3 minutes.

4. Add the garlic, ginger, and sesame seeds and sauté for an additional 5 minutes.

5. Add the bell pepper, corn, water chestnuts, and bamboo shoots and sauté for an additional 3 minutes.

6. Add the cabbage, mushrooms, sprouts, and cilantro and sauté for an additional 3 minutes.

7. Mix the soy sauce, vinegar, agave, broth, and cornstarch in a small dish until smooth. Add to the pan with the vegetables and continue to sauté for about 3 minutes, until the sauce has thickened and the vegetables are crisp-tender. Garnish the stir-fry with the green onions and cashews and serve with the rice.

note: A food processor may come in handy for slicing the fresh vegetables in this recipe.

variation: Add 12 ounces of sliced extra firm tofu (pressed for best results—see page 103) with cabbage.

PER SERVING: 272 calories, 10 g protein, 44 g carbohydrate, 9 g fat, 1.5 g saturated fat, 6 g fiber, 9 g sugar, 279 mg sodium
STAR NUTRIENTS: folate (27% DV), niacin (18% DV), riboflavin (13% DV), thiamin (19% DV), vitamin A (107% DV), vitamin B6 (27% DV), vitamin C (96% DV), vitamin K (68% DV), calcium (14% DV), copper (50% DV), iron (14% DV), magnesium (26% DV), manganese (70% DV), phosphorus (25% DV), potassium (18% DV), selenium (15% DV), zinc (14% DV)

fettuccine with romesco sauce

ACTIVE PREPARATION TIME: 8 minutes • TOTAL PREPARATION TIME: 11 minutes

Romesco sauce was created in northeastern Spain as a flavorful accompaniment for local seafood and vegetable dishes. This rich red sauce is powered by tangy roasted red peppers—packed with disease-fighting lycopene— and served with fresh pasta, which may be found in the refrigerator section of many supermarkets. It's a great dish to launch your plant-powered diet, though you can serve it with a small amount of animal protein, if you're so inclined. Save leftover sauce as a dip for toasted bread.

MAKES 8 SERVINGS
(about ⅔ cup pasta with ⅓ cup Romesco Sauce each)

Romesco Sauce
1 small chile pepper, with seeds, destemmed and sliced into
quarters
3 medium garlic cloves
One 15.5-ounce (439 g) jar roasted red bell peppers, with liquid
½ cup (46 g) toasted sliced almonds
3 tablespoons tomato paste
1 tablespoon smoked paprika
Pinch of cayenne pepper
3 tablespoons red wine vinegar
1 tablespoon extra virgin olive oil
Pinch of sea salt, optional
1 pound (454 g) fresh fettuccine (whole grain if available; see
Notes)

Optional garnishes
Additional toasted almonds
Fresh herb leaves, such as basil, rosemary, or oregano

1. To make the Romesco Sauce: Place the chile pepper, garlic, roasted bell peppers, almonds, tomato paste, paprika, cayenne, vinegar, and olive oil into a food processor or blender and blend until smooth, about 1 minute. Scrape down the sides halfway through blending if necessary. Taste and mix in a pinch of sea salt, if desired.

2. Transfer the Romesco Sauce to a serving bowl and leave at room temperature unless serving it later (see Notes).

3. Bring a large pot of water to a boil and add the fettuccine. Cook for 2 to 3 minutes, just until tender. Drain off the water. Place the fettuccine on

a serving platter and serve immediately, topping individual portions with the Romesco Sauce. Garnish with the additional almonds and fresh herb leaves, if desired.

notes: If you cannot find fresh whole grain fettuccine, you may substitute an equal amount of dried pasta and cook for 8 to 10 minutes, according to the package directions. This recipe is gluten-free if you use gluten-free fettuccine.

Store leftover Romesco Sauce in an airtight container in the refrigerator for up to 2 weeks. It is excellent as a sauce or spread for breads and as an accompaniment to grain salads and vegetables.

variation: Stir 8 ounces of diced baked tofu or seitan into the prepared Romesco Sauce before serving.

PER SERVING: 297 calories, 11 g protein, 51 g carbohydrate, 7 g fat, 1 g saturated fat, 9 g fiber, 2 g sugar, 144 mg sodium
STAR NUTRIENTS: folate (10% DV), niacin (17% DV), riboflavin (11% DV), thiamin (20% DV), vitamin A (19% DV), vitamin B6 (10% DV), vitamin C (35% DV), vitamin E (14% DV), copper (18% DV), iron (20% DV), magnesium (27% DV), manganese (99% DV), phosphorus (20% DV), zinc (11% DV)

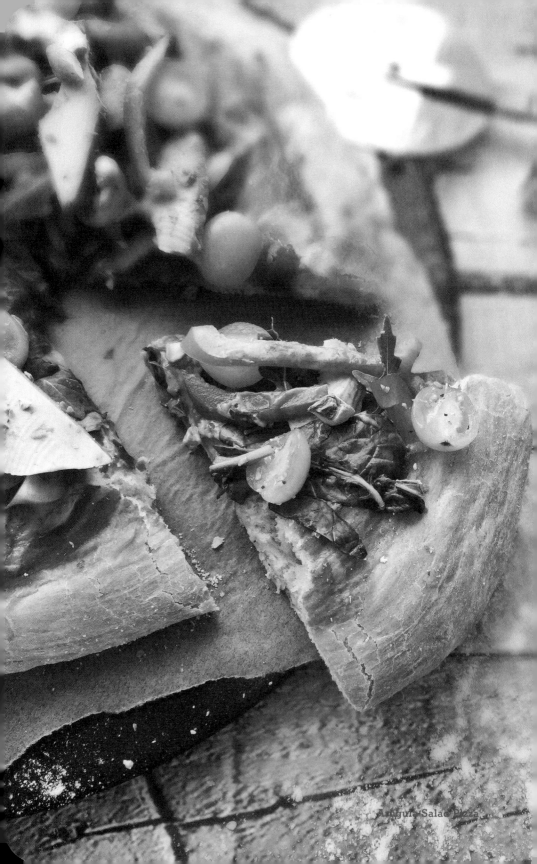

Take meat off the center of your plate.

Tofu Mushroom Tacos
Arugula Salad Pizza
Chickpea Stew with Kale and Za'atar

Picture this: an oversize dinner plate with a big piece of meat in the center, a scoop of mashed potatoes on the side, and an even smaller scoop of green beans on the other side. Or this: a fast-food tray with a double cheeseburger on a white bun, a piece of wilted lettuce and a slice of tomato on the side, and an overflowing cone of french fries. In both meals, animal foods—especially meat—are at the center of the plate, with a skimpy side showing of (often processed) plant foods.

These meals represent the typical American diet, which your parents— and maybe you—learned is "healthy." It's the sort of meal planning that has pushed America to consume three times the global rate of meat. It's also what has us on the fast track for obesity, heart disease, type 2 diabetes, and cancer.

Now picture this: rustic red beans poured over rice beside a mound of simmered squash, peppers, onions, and herbs. Or whole grain pita bread served with hummus, a bulgur mint salad, and a generous portion of roasted eggplant. These meals focus on local, seasonal produce and treat meat—if it's used at all—as a seasoning, not the main event. Around the world—from Africa to South America to Asia—people who eat this way tend to suffer from lower rates of chronic disease. Scientists have dubbed these eating styles "poor man's" diets, but they are often rich in both taste and nutrition.

One of the easiest ways to transition to a plant-powered diet is to shift your thinking about meal planning. When you plan your menu for the week, don't think of chicken on Monday and beef on Tuesday; think of kale on Monday and lentils on Tuesday. Start with the plants, and you won't miss the meat.

tofu mushroom tacos

ACTIVE PREPARATION TIME: **17 minutes** • TOTAL PREPARATION TIME: **17 minutes**

It's easy to move away from the "meat as the center of the plate" attitude when you focus on fresh, globally inspired dishes, like these spicy tacos. You won't even miss the beef when you cook up this quick dish, sure to please the entire family. Pair it with Tortilla Soup (page 112) to balance out your meal. Best of all: save leftover taco filling and reheat for a speedy, easy lunch the next day.

MAKES 8 SERVINGS
(1 taco each)

8 ounces (227 g) extra firm tofu, drained and pressed for best results (see page 103)
1 teaspoon extra virgin olive oil
1½ cups (105 g) finely chopped mushrooms (e.g., white, baby portobello)
2 green onions, white and green parts, diced
1 medium garlic clove, minced
2 tablespoons prepared salsa, plus ½ cup (130 g) for serving
1 teaspoon low-sodium taco seasoning (see page 345)
1 teaspoon reduced sodium soy sauce
One 15-ounce (425 g) can black beans, no salt added, rinsed and drained (or 1¾ cups cooked)
2 cups (72 g) packed leafy greens
2 medium tomatoes, diced
1 medium avocado, peeled, cored, and sliced into 8 pieces
Eight 6-inch (23 g) whole grain tortillas (e.g., corn, whole wheat)
1 cup (112 g) shredded plant-based cheese, optional
Plant-based sour cream (see page 344), optional

1. Shred the tofu with a grater or in a food processor (with shredding attachment).
2. Heat the olive oil in a large skillet over medium heat and add the shredded tofu, mushrooms, green onions, and garlic. Sauté for 2 minutes.
3. Add the salsa, taco seasoning, and soy sauce. Sauté for an additional 5 to 7 minutes, until the mushrooms are tender.
4. Meanwhile, heat the black beans in the microwave or on the stovetop over medium heat until warm.
5. Arrange the greens, tomatoes, and avocado on a platter.
6. Warm the tortillas in the microwave or in a hot skillet for 30 seconds.

7. To assemble the tacos: Fill each tortilla with about ¼ cup of the tofu-mushroom mixture, ¼ cup of black beans, ¼ cup of greens, 3 tablespoons chopped tomato, 1 slice of avocado, 2 tablespoons of plant-based cheese, a dollop of plant-based sour cream (if desired), and 1 tablespoon of salsa.

note: Store the leftover taco filling in an airtight container in the refrigerator for up to 2 days. Reheat for a few minutes in the microwave or a small skillet and serve with the remaining ingredients, as suggested.

PER SERVING: 244 calories, 10 g protein, 31 g carbohydrate, 10 g fat, 2 g saturated fat, 7 g fiber, 2 g sugar, 430 mg sodium
STAR NUTRIENTS: folate (13% DV), vitamin A (11% DV), vitamin C (14% DV), vitamin K (13% DV), calcium (13% DV), iron (11% DV), potassium (12% DV)

See photo
on page 6

arugula salad pizza

ACTIVE PREPARATION TIME: **13 minutes** • TOTAL PREPARATION TIME: **45 minutes**

Here's how you rethink your plate: a fresh green salad and whole grain pizza all in one meal that you can whip up in 45 minutes. Now that's quick and delicious eating for even the busiest night of your week! Pair it with my hearty Red Lentil Soup with Root Vegetables and Sage (page 178) for a completely satisfying meal.

MAKES 8 SERVINGS
(1 slice each)

Whole grain pizza dough (see Notes), or one 16-ounce (454 g) package refrigerated whole grain pizza dough, or whole grain pizza dough prepared from a mix
Cornmeal for sprinkling
⅓ cup (86 g) marinara sauce
1½ teaspoons dried oregano
1 cup (112 g) shredded plant-based cheese (see Notes)
2 cups (62 g) mixed fresh arugula and baby spinach
1½ cups (224 g) fresh yellow cherry tomatoes, halved
½ medium red bell pepper, diced
1 ripe medium avocado, sliced
¼ cup (31 g) roasted pistachios
1 tablespoon balsamic vinegar
1 tablespoon extra virgin olive oil

1. Preheat the oven to 350°F (180°C). Roll out the pizza dough to fit a 14-inch pizza pan or pizza stone. Sprinkle the pan or stone with cornmeal and fit the dough on top.
2. Spread the marinara sauce onto the dough and sprinkle the oregano and plant-based cheese over it. Place the pan or stone in the oven and bake for 30 to 35 minutes, until the crust is golden and firm to the touch.
3. At the last minute before serving, remove the crust from the oven and top with the arugula and spinach, tomatoes, bell pepper, avocado, and pistachios. The greens will wilt quickly.
4. Drizzle with the vinegar and olive oil. Serve immediately.

notes: You may prepare your own pizza dough following this procedure: Stir together ¾ cup warm (110°F/43°C) water, 1½ teaspoons active dry yeast, and 1 teaspoon honey in a medium bowl. Let stand for 10 minutes. Stir in 1½ teaspoons extra virgin olive oil and 1¾ cups whole wheat flour. Tip the dough onto a lightly floured surface and knead for 10 minutes. Place the dough in an oiled bowl, cover with a towel, and let it rise in a warm place for about 1 hour, then proceed with step 1 of the recipe.

Omit the plant-based cheese, if desired.

variation: Substitute other firm greens, such as baby kale or chopped collard greens, for the arugula and baby spinach.

PER SERVING: 258 calories, 12 g protein, 34 g carbohydrate, 8 g fat, 1 g saturated fat, 5 g fiber, 5 g sugar, 466 mg sodium
STAR NUTRIENTS: vitamin A (11% DV), vitamin C (28% DV), vitamin K (19% DV), calcium (15% DV), iron (11% DV)

chickpea stew with kale and za'atar

ACTIVE PREPARATION TIME: **13 minutes** • TOTAL PREPARATION TIME: **17 minutes**

One surefire way to create a plant-centric plate is to focus on Mediterranean foods—quintessential plant-based fare linked with a plethora of benefits. This Mediterranean dish gets its kick from za'atar, a traditional Middle Eastern seasoning mix, which includes sumac, thyme, sesame seeds, marjoram, and oregano. Often sprinkled on top of prepared foods for extra flavor, za'atar gives this easy stew—you can prepare it in minutes—its vibrant flavor. Serve it with whole grain pita and Muhammara (page 177).

MAKES 8 SERVINGS
(generous 1 cup each)

1 teaspoon extra virgin olive oil
1 small onion, diced
2 medium garlic cloves, minced
2½ teaspoons za'atar (see Note)
½ teaspoon crushed red pepper
One 14.5-ounce (411 g) can diced tomatoes, no salt added, with
     juice
One 15-ounce (425 g) can chickpeas, no salt added, rinsed and
     drained (or 1¾ cups cooked)
2 cups (474 ml) water
1 teaspoon reduced sodium vegetable broth base
10 ounces (283 g) chopped fresh kale (about 4 cups)
Juice of ½ lemon

1. Heat the olive oil in a medium pot over medium heat. Add the onion, garlic, za'atar, and crushed red pepper and sauté over medium heat for about 2 minutes.

2. Add the tomatoes, chickpeas, water, and broth base, cover the pot, and bring to a boil over medium-high heat.

3. Stir the kale and lemon juice into the boiling liquid, reduce the heat to medium, and cook for about 2 minutes, until the kale is just wilted but still bright green.

4. Serve immediately.

note: You can find za'atar in a Middle Eastern or Mediterranean shop or gourmet food store. To make your own, see page 345.

PER SERVING: 116 calories, 6 g protein, 19 g carbohydrate, 2 g fat, 0 g saturated fat, 4 g fiber, 2 g sugar, 187 mg sodium
STAR NUTRIENTS: folate (10% DV), vitamin A (75% DV), vitamin C (87% DV), vitamin K (313% DV), calcium (10% DV), copper (34% DV), manganese (36% DV), potassium (10% DV)

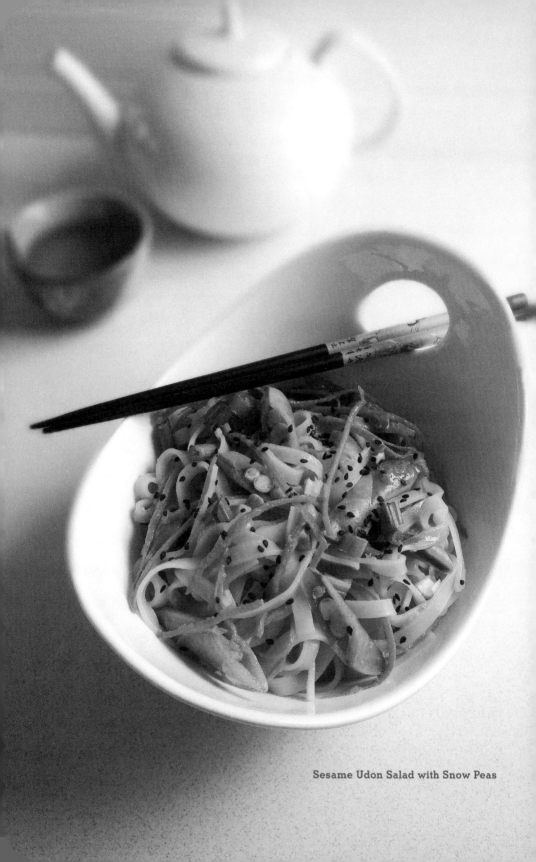

Sesame Udon Salad with Snow Peas

Reclaim your culinary traditions, or develop new ones.

Green Bean Casserole with Caramelized Onions
Red Bean and Okra Jambalaya
Sesame Udon Salad with Snow Peas

❦

Many of us already eat food from a wide variety of culinary traditions: One night, we might eat curry, and the next, a burrito. Global inspiration can be delicious and healthful (see page 117), but when variety comes only from eating out, we consume far more calories, fat, saturated fat, sugar, and sodium than we need. And we miss out on sustaining (or creating) our own food traditions.

From the very beginning, humans shared resources, protection, and food in exchange for the well-being of the individual and the community. By now, it's in our DNA to share food. It offers so much more than mere physical sustenance; it provides pleasure, warmth, love, joy, celebration, and nurturing. It's why all of the best moments in life—weddings, religious events, anniversaries, birthdays—are marked with the sharing of food.

Over the centuries, children learned about their food culture in kitchens with their parents, and they passed this knowledge down to the next generation. Perhaps a young girl learned to cook greens—the perfect way to wash, roll, slice, and cook them—with her mother, a tradition that might have been traced back to West Africa generations ago. All it takes is one link to be broken, and that family tradition is lost forever.

I have my own view of food traditions, filtered through my mother's upbringing in Arkansas, my father's in Minnesota, our family's (nearly) vegetarian commitment, and my childhood in the Pacific Northwest. My swirl of food memories include the sweet smell of ripe strawberries on a Washington berry farm, my mom's savory pots of black-eyed peas, and my dad's "Johnny cake" (cornbread). Dig into your own memories to resurrect your cultural food traditions. These traditions might be rooted in the country of your ancestors, or even the region you grew up in. They may include facets of religion, celebrations, family events, holidays, and weekends.

What are the food traditions you will celebrate and pass on to your friends and family?

green bean casserole with caramelized onions

ACTIVE PREPARATION TIME: **16 minutes** • TOTAL PREPARATION TIME: **40 minutes**

Get in touch with your culinary roots by looking to the favorite foods of your past. For many, those roots include classic American comfort foods, like a piping hot green bean casserole, fresh from the oven. My plant-powered version, which swaps mounds of golden, caramelized onions for processed, deep-fried onions, is just as healthful as it is delicious.

MAKES 6 SERVINGS
(about ¾ cup each)

1 tablespoon extra virgin olive oil
1 large yellow onion, halved and sliced into rings
¼ teaspoon freshly ground black pepper
4 cups (948 ml) water
1 pound (454 g) fresh green beans, trimmed (see Note)
5 ounces (142 g) sliced fresh white mushrooms (2 cups)
2 medium garlic cloves, minced
¼ teaspoon sweet paprika
¼ teaspoon nutmeg
2 tablespoons all purpose flour, or 1 tablespoon cornstarch for
    gluten-free
1½ cups (355 ml) unsweetened plant-based milk (e.g., soy,
    almond, coconut milk beverage)
Pinch of sea salt, optional
2 tablespoons whole grain bread crumbs
    (see Note on page 95)

1. Heat ½ tablespoon of the olive oil in a skillet or sauté pan over medium heat, then add the onion and black pepper. Sauté for 9 to 10 minutes, until the onion rings are caramelized and brown. Remove the onions from the skillet and set aside, reserving the empty skillet.

2. Meanwhile, heat the water in a large pot and add the green beans. Cover and cook for 5 minutes. Drain the beans and place them in a 2-quart casserole dish.

3. Preheat the oven to 375°F (190°C).

4. Heat ½ tablespoon of the olive oil in the same skillet used for the onions. Add the mushrooms, garlic, paprika, and nutmeg and sauté for 4 minutes.

5. Whisk the flour and plant-based milk together in a small dish until smooth with no lumps. Stir into the mushroom mixture and cook for about

1 minute, until the mixture thickens. Season with a pinch of sea salt, if desired. Pour the mushroom sauce into the casserole dish with the green beans and stir well.

6. Top the green bean mixture with the onions and bread crumbs. Bake uncovered for 20 minutes and serve piping hot.

note: You may replace the fresh green beans with frozen (thawed) or canned (no salt added, drained) green beans. Skip cooking the beans (as in step 2) and add them directly to the casserole dish.

PER SERVING: 110 calories, 7 g protein, 15 g carbohydrate, 4 g fat, .5 g saturated fat, 4 g fiber, 5 g sugar, 80 mg sodium
STAR NUTRIENTS: folate (10% DV), riboflavin (14% DV), vitamin A (14% DV), vitamin B6 (11% DV), vitamin C (21% DV), vitamin K (14% DV), calcium (13% DV), manganese (13% DV)

red bean and okra jambalaya

ACTIVE PREPARATION TIME: **18 minutes** • TOTAL PREPARATION TIME: **1 hour 30 minutes**

No matter where you're from, you can borrow from the culinary melting pot of the world in order to infuse your plate with a bold essence. The Creole flavors of New Orleans—steeped in a rich tradition of cultures, including African, Caribbean, and the New World—are among my favorites. You might be surprised to discover that many of these traditional dishes, such as jambalaya, are based on plant foods: beans and rice. This one-pot meal is bursting with flavor; serve it with a crusty whole wheat baguette for a hearty meal. And the leftovers are wonderful the next day.

MAKES 6 SERVINGS
(about 1½ cups each)

1 teaspoon extra virgin olive oil
1 large onion, diced
3 medium garlic cloves, minced
¼ teaspoon cayenne pepper
¼ teaspoon sweet paprika
¼ teaspoon cumin
2 teaspoons chili powder
¼ teaspoon celery salt
Hot sauce, optional
1 cup (200 g) uncooked short-grain brown rice
2 medium bell peppers (red, orange, green, or yellow), diced
2 medium carrots, sliced
2 celery stalks, sliced
2 cups (200 g) chopped fresh or frozen okra
One 14.5-ounce (411 g) can fire-roasted diced tomatoes, with juice
One 15-ounce (425 g) can red beans, no salt added, with liquid
    (or 1¾ cups cooked, with ⅔ cup water)
2 cups (474 ml) reduced sodium vegetable broth (see page 346)
½ cup (119 ml) water
¼ cup (15 g) chopped fresh parsley

1. Heat the olive oil in a large skillet over medium heat.
2. Add the onions and cook for 5 minutes.
3. Add the garlic, cayenne, paprika, cumin, chili powder, celery salt, hot sauce (if desired), and rice. Cook for 2 minutes, stirring often.
4. Add the bell peppers, carrots, celery, and okra. Sauté for an additional 5 minutes, stirring frequently.
5. Add the tomatoes, red beans, broth, and water. Stir well. Bring to a boil, reduce the heat to medium-low, cover, and cook for 1 hour and 10 to 20

minutes, until the rice is tender, stirring frequently. Add additional water as needed to compensate for moisture lost to evaporation, but avoid thinning the consistency too much (it should be thick).

6. Remove from the heat and sprinkle with the parsley immediately before serving.

variation: Substitute any other kind of bean for the red beans (such as black beans, chickpeas, or heirloom varieties).

PER SERVING: 280 calories, 10 g protein, 56 g carbohydrates, 3 g fat, 1 g saturated fat, 12 g fiber, 7 g sugar, 424 mg sodium
STAR NUTRIENTS: folate (17% DV), thiamin (11% DV), vitamin A (110% DV), vitamin B6 (15% DV), vitamin C (113% DV), vitamin K (74% DV), calcium (12% DV), copper (15% DV), iron (16% DV), magnesium (13% DV), manganese (35% DV), phosphorus (14% DV), potassium (19% DV), zinc (12% DV

See photo on page 14

sesame udon salad with snow peas

ACTIVE PREPARATION TIME: **20 minutes** • TOTAL PREPARATION TIME: **20 minutes**

Call upon a traditional Asian cooking flair to power your meals with potent flavor and health. Packed with a variety of flavors, textures, and colors, this easy Japanese-inspired salad can be whipped up in mere minutes. It's an excellent dish to tote along to a potluck or to the office in your lunch box. As the flavors meld together, it's even better the next day.

MAKES 6 SERVINGS
(generous 1 cup each)

9.5 ounces (260 g) dried udon noodles
1 tablespoon rice vinegar
2 tablespoons orange juice
1 tablespoon honey or agave nectar
3 tablespoons reduced sodium soy sauce
1 tablespoon sesame oil
1 tablespoon unsalted creamy peanut butter
½ teaspoon minced fresh ginger
2 medium garlic cloves, minced
¼ teaspoon crushed red pepper
8 ounces (227 g) fresh snow peas, trimmed and halved
1 medium carrot, sliced into small matchsticks
3 green onions, white and green parts, sliced
1 tablespoon sesame seeds (black or beige)

1. Bring a medium pot of water to a boil. Add the udon noodles and cook, uncovered, for about 10 minutes (according to package directions). Place in a colander and rinse with cold water, draining off the liquid.

2. In a small dish, make the dressing by whisking together the vinegar, orange juice, honey, soy sauce, sesame oil, peanut butter, ginger, garlic, and crushed red pepper.

3. Transfer the rinsed, cooled noodles to a large mixing bowl. Add the dressing and toss. Add the snow peas, carrot, and green onions and toss again. Sprinkle with the sesame seeds.

4. Chill until serving time.

variations: Add 8 ounces (227 g) of cubed tofu (pressed, for best results—see page 103) or one 15-ounce (425 g) can (1¾ cups) of drained and rinsed, no salt added beans, such as adzuki or kidney, in step 3.

Use rice noodles instead of the udon noodles to make this gluten-free.

PER SERVING: 230 calories, 9 g protein, 40 g carbohydrate, 4.5 g fat, .5 g saturated fat, 3 g fiber, 7 g sugar, 315 mg sodium
STAR NUTRIENTS: niacin (11% DV), thiamin (10% DV), vitamin A (38% DV), vitamin C (48% DV), iron (13% DV)

French Lentil Salad
with Cherry Tomatoes

Love your legumes for protein and beyond.

Caribbean Calypso Beans
French Lentil Salad with Cherry Tomatoes

Ah, the humble bean. Legumes, which are seeds harvested from their pods when mature, including dried beans, peas, and lentils, are staples in just about every traditional diet around the globe, from chickpeas in the Middle East to red beans in Central America. And for good reason, too—these economical, nonperishable plant foods are about as near to perfection as you can get. A half-cup serving provides a good supply of at least nine essential vitamins and minerals, as well as a hefty dose of fiber, slow-digesting carbs, and protein. In fact, a half-cup serving of cooked legumes has about the same amount of protein as an ounce of meat, so you can see why it's important to include these gems every day in your plant-powered diet.

Legumes are also rich in plant-protective phytochemicals linked with health protection. For example, many dark-colored legumes, such as black beans and black ("beluga") lentils, contain anthocyanins, the same health-promoting pigments found in many brightly colored berries, such as blueberries and cranberries. Today, many of us fall short on our intake of these healthy plant foods; they have been supplanted by animal foods and highly processed products in our modern diet.

Plan to make a return to legumes every day. For breakfast, try pinto, kidney, or black beans with whole grain tortillas or even baked beans on toast, English-style. Savor a bean or lentil chili or hummus wrap for lunch, and serve a simmered bean curry or stewed black-eyed peas with greens for dinner. Beans can even be part of snack time, if you nibble on edamame straight from the pod or roast some whole chickpeas in spices (see page 30). To help avoid digestive upset, introduce legumes to your diet slowly if you're unused to them, but eventually shoot for at least one serving a day for optimal health benefits.

caribbean calypso beans

ACTIVE PREPARATION TIME: **18 minutes** • TOTAL PREPARATION TIME: **1 hour 45 minutes**
(not including soaking time)

Try to include beans in your diet at least a few times a week. It's not hard, when there are so many delicious, colorful varieties. Beautiful heirloom calypso beans—with their dark swirl against pale flesh—are the perfect blank canvas for a Caribbean-inspired recipe. Look for calypso beans in natural food stores or online. If you can't find them, simply use kidney beans in this vibrant dish. Serve these beans with whole grain tortillas and salad greens for a hearty, wholesome meal.

MAKES 10 SERVINGS
(about 1 cup each)

12 ounces (340 g or about 1¾ cups) dried calypso beans
    or kidney beans
2 cups (474 ml) water, plus more for soaking
2 cups (474 ml) reduced sodium vegetable broth (see page 346)
½ cup (119 ml) orange juice
One 6-ounce (170 g) can tomato paste
1 teaspoon extra virgin olive oil
1 medium onion, diced
1 medium red bell pepper, diced
1 medium jalapeño pepper, finely diced
2 medium garlic cloves, minced
½ teaspoon coriander
½ teaspoon cumin
1 teaspoon thyme
¼ teaspoon smoked paprika (may adjust according to desired
    preference)
10 saffron threads, crushed (with mortar and pestle)
1 bay leaf
½ cup (30 g) chopped fresh cilantro

1. Cover the beans with water and soak overnight.
2. Drain the beans and add to a large pot with the 2 cups of water, broth, orange juice, and tomato paste. Cover and bring to a boil over medium-high heat and reduce the heat to medium and cook for a total of 1½ hours.
3. While the beans are cooking, heat the olive oil in a skillet. Add the onion and sauté for 4 minutes. Add the bell pepper, jalapeño, garlic, coriander, cumin, thyme, and paprika and sauté for 4 additional minutes. Add the sautéed vegetable mixture, saffron, and bay leaf to the pot of beans and cover.

4. Stir the beans occasionally, adding water as needed to replace moisture lost to evaporation, although the consistency should be thick. When the beans are tender (after about 1½ hours total cooking time), remove the bay leaf and top with fresh cilantro.

note: To prepare this dish in a slow cooker, place the soaked beans and all remaining ingredients into the slow cooker and cook on high for 4 to 5 hours. For best results, sauté the vegetables as indicated in step 3 before adding them to the slow cooker.

PER SERVING: 153 calories, 10 g protein, 28 g carbohydrate, 1 g fat, 0 g saturated fat, 10 g fiber, 5 g sugar, 257 mg sodium
STAR NUTRIENTS: folate (37% DV), thiamin (15% DV), vitamin B6 (12% DV), vitamin C (79% DV), vitamin K (15% DV), copper (21% DV), iron (20% DV), magnesium (15% DV), manganese (23% DV), phosphorus (16% DV), potassium (23% DV)

See photo
on page 22

french lentil salad with cherry tomatoes

ACTIVE PREPARATION TIME: **15 minutes** • TOTAL PREPARATION TIME: **30 minutes**
(not including chilling time)

Beans aren't the only member of the legume family worth celebrating. Lentils, packed with fiber and protein, are just as nutritious. Plus they cook up—no soaking required—in only 15 to 20 minutes. A French ami shared her mother's traditional recipe for lentil salad with me years ago. This simple salad, seasoned with a French vinaigrette, is a classic dish in France. It makes a wonderful, protein-rich highlight of any meal. Because the flavors continue to meld, it's also great the next day. Serve it with toasted whole wheat French bread and Tofu Ratatouille (page 250) for a true country French meal.

MAKES 6 SERVINGS
(about 1 cup each)

1 pound (454 g) dried lentils (or 3 cups cooked; see Note)
4 cups (948 ml) water
2 teaspoons reduced sodium vegetable broth base
4 celery stalks, diced (160 g or about 1½ cups)
1½ cups (224 g) cherry tomatoes, halved
2 medium shallots, finely diced
¼ cup (15 g) packed chopped fresh parsley
1½ tablespoons extra virgin olive oil
2 teaspoons Dijon mustard
2 tablespoons red wine vinegar
1 teaspoon herbes de Provence (see page 345)
Freshly ground black pepper, to taste
1 medium garlic clove, minced
Pinch of sea salt, optional

1. Place the lentils, water, and broth base in a pot. Cover and bring to a boil over medium-high heat. Reduce the heat to medium and cook for 15 to 20 minutes, until the lentils are tender but firm.

2. Remove from the heat, drain any remaining liquid, and transfer the lentils to a large bowl. Chill for at least 30 minutes.

3. Stir in the celery, tomatoes, shallots, and parsley.

4. In a small dish, make the dressing by whisking together the olive oil, mustard, vinegar, herbes de Provence, black pepper, and garlic.

5. Add the dressing to the lentil mixture and toss. Taste and season with sea salt, if desired. Chill until serving time.

note: If you're in a rush, use precooked, refrigerated lentils, available at many stores. Although a classic French lentil salad uses *lentils du puys* (small, dark green lentils), try other varieties for a colorful twist, such as yellow, beluga (black), or multicolored lentils.

variation: Substitute cooked beans, such as white, fava, or cranberry beans, for the lentils.

PER SERVING: 136 calories, 8 g protein, 19 g carbohydrate, 4 g fat, .5 g saturated fat, 4 g fiber, 3 g sugar, 55 mg sodium
STAR NUTRIENTS: folate (40% DV), thiamin (10% DV), vitamin A (13% DV), vitamin B6 (11% DV), vitamin C (19% DV), vitamin K (67% DV), copper (13% DV), iron (16% DV), magnesium (10% DV), manganese (24% DV), phosphorus (16% DV), potassium (14% DV)

Haricots Verts, Tomato, and
Almond Salad

Choose foods as close to nature as possible.

Roasted Chickpeas with Spices
Haricots Verts, Tomato, and Almond Salad

*W*hole foods: it's a term on everyone's tongue (and I'm not referring to the supermarket chain!). But what *is* a whole food? Think of it as "close to nature." Seeing a whole food up close, you can imagine how the food was grown. For example, when I see a bunch of mustard greens, I think of that plant, with its roots pushed into the soil, and envision the farmer snipping off the crisp green leaves at the base of the plant. The same thing happens when I see a bulk bin of white beans. I think of the trailing bean vine pushing forth long bean pods in the warm sun, and of the farmer allowing the seeds to mature and dry in the pods before harvesting them.

Foods such as these are purchased "whole"—they are not pulverized, chemically refined, or denatured. They do not require food labels or marketing slogans at the supermarket. We simply take them home, wash them, cook them, and eat them. Yet, so many plant foods on shelves have endured countless modifications before they are packaged into foods. For example, grains are stripped of their nutrient-rich coverings; other ingredients are refined until they bear no resemblance to the plant from which they came. If you can't recognize the plant that gave birth to your food, chances are you're losing out on the nutrients—fiber, vitamins, minerals, phytochemicals— found in their flesh, skins, and seeds.

Try to make sure *most* of your foods are as close to nature as possible. Look for foods that are real and minimally processed—with ingredients that you can see with the naked eye. Think carrots, not orange snack puffs; almonds, not almond-flavored nutrition bars; lentils, not lentil chips.

roasted chickpeas with spices

ACTIVE PREPARATION TIME: **15 minutes** • TOTAL PREPARATION TIME: **1 hour 30 minutes**
(not including soaking time)

When it comes to variety, don't stop at mealtime—your snacks are a wonderful opportunity to power up on flavorful whole plant foods. And if you're looking for an aromatic, exotically spiced, healthy snack option, look no further. These roasted chickpeas are bursting with addictive flavor and crunch. Set out a bowl of them as an appetizer at a party, or make a batch to enjoy as snacks throughout the week. Each serving is packed with 7 grams of protein and 7 grams of fiber, meaning that this snack will help keep you feeling full and satisfied until your next meal.

MAKES 12 SERVINGS
(about ½ cup each)

1 pound (448 g) dried chickpeas
¼ teaspoon crushed red pepper (see Notes)
3 cardamom pods
¼ teaspoon fenugreek seeds
½ teaspoon cumin seeds
¼ teaspoon coriander seeds
¼ teaspoon mustard seeds
2 tablespoons extra virgin olive oil
Juice of 1 medium lemon
2 medium garlic cloves, minced
Pinch of sea salt, optional

1. Place the chickpeas in a large bowl, cover with water, and soak overnight.
2. Drain the chickpeas and return to the bowl.
3. Preheat the oven to 375°F (190°C).
4. Place all of the spices in a blender or small food processor. Process for about 1 minute, until the spices are finely ground.
5. Add the olive oil, lemon juice, and garlic to the spices and process until the garlic is chopped and all ingredients are well combined.
6. Add the spice mixture to the chickpeas and toss to coat well.
7. Spread the chickpeas in a layer on a large baking sheet and place in the oven. Bake for about 1 hour and 15 minutes—depending on your own preference for crispness—stirring every 15 minutes.
8. Serve immediately, sprinkled with sea salt, if desired.

notes: You may store the chickpeas in the refrigerator for up to 3 days. These are best served warm—you may reheat briefly in the microwave to freshen them.

If you prefer a spicier snack, increase the amount of crushed red pepper.

PER SERVING: 161 calories, 7 g protein, 24 g carbohydrate, 5 g fat, .5 g saturated fat, 7 g fiber, 4 g sugar, 4 mg sodium
STAR NUTRIENTS: folate (53% DV), thiamin (13% DV), vitamin B6 (11% DV), iron (14% DV), magnesium (11% DV), potassium (10% DV)

See photo
on page 28

haricots verts, tomato,
and almond salad

ACTIVE PREPARATION TIME: 10 minutes • TOTAL PREPARATION TIME: 30 minutes

It's easy to see Mother Nature's hand in this classic French green bean salad. Thin, tender green beans—ideally haricots verts, a French variety—form the core of this salad tossed with a traditional French vinaigrette. These simple emerald beauties are bursting with fiber, vitamins, minerals and phytochemicals in the carotenoid family—nutrients linked with heart health. If you're interested in trying your hand at a vegetable garden, the lovely canopy of haricots verts vines growing on a trellis might make this a fun plant to start with.

MAKES 6 SERVINGS
(about 1¼ cups each)

2 cups (474 ml) water
8 ounces (227 g) thin green beans, preferably haricots verts,
    trimmed
Juice of ½ lemon
1 tablespoon extra virgin olive oil
1 teaspoon honey or agave nectar
1 teaspoon Dijon mustard
1 teaspoon thyme
1 medium garlic clove, minced
Pinch of freshly ground black pepper
Pinch of sea salt, optional
3 cups (141 g) packed baby greens, such as romaine, arugula,
    or leaf lettuce
2 medium tomatoes, chopped
3 tablespoons coarsely chopped toasted almonds, preferably
    Marcona

1. Place the water in a medium pot and bring it to a boil. Add the green beans, cover, and cook on medium heat for 6 minutes. Drain the beans and transfer to a small bowl.

2. Meanwhile, make the dressing by whisking together the lemon juice, olive oil, honey, mustard, thyme, garlic, black pepper, and sea salt, if desired. Pour the dressing over the green beans and place in the refrigerator to marinate for about 20 minutes.

3. Line a platter with the greens.

4. Add the tomatoes to the chilled green beans and toss. Arrange the mixture over the greens and sprinkle with the almonds.

note: If you are making this salad ahead of time, it will keep well stored in an airtight container in the refrigerator for up to 3 days. Add the lettuce and almonds at the last moment to keep from wilting and turning soft.

PER SERVING: 69 calories, 2 g protein, 6 g carbohydrate, 4 g fat, .5 g saturated fat, 2 g fiber, 3 g sugar, 18 mg sodium
STAR NUTRIENTS: folate (10% DV), vitamin A (49% DV), vitamin C (14% DV), vitamin K (34% DV)

Farro and White Bean
Veggie Burgers

Collect a plant-powered pantry arsenal.

Farro and White Bean Veggie Burgers
Steel-Cut Oats Risotto with Asparagus

If you don't have all of the essential ingredients on hand for living la vida plant-powered, then it simply won't happen! You will be forever running to the store, or simply giving up on wholesome plant-based meals altogether. Yet, this style of eating can be easy, breezy if you just power up your pantry with shelf-stable plant foods: whole grains, legumes, spices, nuts, and seeds.

Once you have the essentials on hand, all you have to do is supplement with fresh ingredients—vegetables, fruits, tofu, plant-based milks—to turn out fabulous meals in mere minutes. A bag of brown rice is the foundation for a stir-fry, a pouch of garbanzos can kick-start a curry, and steel-cut oats form the cornerstone of breakfast cereal, as well as risotto (see Steel-Cut Oats Risotto with Asparagus on page 38).

Keep these pantry basics on hand at all times:

- **Dried or canned beans, peas, and lentils,** such as kidney beans, chickpeas, black-eyed peas, and lentils
- **Canned, frozen, or dried vegetables,** such as canned tomatoes, frozen green peas, dried sea vegetables (see Note on page 132), and sun-dried tomatoes
- **Canned, frozen, or dried fruits,** such as canned unsweetened peaches and pears and dried, unsweetened fruit, like apples, apricots, and blueberries
- **Herbs and spices,** such as allspice, basil, bay leaves, cardamom, cayenne, cilantro, cumin, garlic, oregano, paprika, parsley, and thyme
- **Nuts and seeds,** such as almonds, peanuts, and flaxseeds
- **Oils,** such as extra virgin olive oil and expeller-pressed canola oil
- **Whole grains,** such as amaranth, bulgur, wheat berries, quinoa, and whole grain flours and pasta

These foods are the start to hundreds of magical, plant-powered meals, from Red Bean and Okra Jambalaya (page 18) to Polenta with Puttanesca Sauce (page 84).

farro and white bean veggie burgers

ACTIVE PREPARATION TIME: 29 minutes • TOTAL PREPARATION TIME: 2½ hours
(including chilling time)

If you stock your plant-powered pantry wisely, you'll be able to pull out fabulous meals every night of the week. Just combine a few staples— canned beans, dried farro, oats, walnuts, herbs, and olive oil—with a few fresh items, including mushrooms, carrots, tomatoes, avocados, and whole grain buns, and you'll have an amazing meal worthy of a special week-night, weekend party, or celebration. Homemade veggie burgers, such as these savory farro and white bean burgers, are leaps and bounds above frozen varieties when it comes to taste. And they're not as hard to make as you think. Make up this big batch for a large group, or to reheat for lunches and meals during the week.

MAKES 10 SERVINGS
(1 patty, bun, and lettuce leaf, and 2 tomato and avocado slices each)

¾ cup (156 g) uncooked farro
3 cups (711 ml) water
1 teaspoon reduced sodium vegetable broth base
One 15-ounce (425 g) can cannellini beans, no salt added,
  rinsed and drained (liquid reserved), or 1¾ cups cooked
1 medium onion, finely diced
1 cup (70 g) finely chopped mushrooms
1 cup (110 g) grated carrots (2 medium)
¼ cup (29 g) chopped walnuts
¼ cup (15 g) chopped fresh oregano, or 1 teaspoon dried
2 tablespoons minced fresh chives
⅓ cup (52 g) uncooked old-fashioned oats
½ cup whole grain bread crumbs (see Note on page 95)
1 teaspoon low-sodium herbal seasoning blend (see page 345)
¼ teaspoon freshly ground black pepper
¼ teaspoon turmeric
Pinch of sea salt, optional
3 tablespoons extra virgin olive oil
Ten 1½-ounce (43 g) whole grain buns
10 lettuce leaves
3 medium tomatoes, sliced into 20 slices
2 avocados, sliced into 20 slices

1. Place the farro in a pot with the water and broth base. Stir well, cover, and bring to a boil over medium-high heat. Reduce the heat to medium, cook for 35 to 40 minutes, and drain any leftover liquid.
2. Place the cannellini beans in a mixing bowl and mash slightly with

a potato masher, until thick and lumpy. Mix in the cooked farro, onions, mushrooms, carrots, walnuts, oregano, chives, oats, bread crumbs, herbal seasoning, black pepper, turmeric, and sea salt, if desired. Combine the ingredients using clean hands, then add 2 to 3 tablespoons of the reserved bean liquid to make a thick yet moistened mixture that sticks together. Chill for about 1 hour.

3. In a large skillet, heat 1 tablespoon of the olive oil over medium heat. Form patties out of ½ cup of the bean mixture with your hands, mashing the ingredients together so that they do not crumble. Carefully place 3 to 4 patties at a time into the hot oil and cook for 6 minutes on each side, turning carefully. Repeat, adding 1 tablespoon of olive oil to the skillet with each batch of patties, until all the patties are done.

4. Serve each patty with 1 bun, 1 lettuce leaf, 2 tomato slices, and 2 avocado slices.

note: If you don't want to serve all of the burgers at once, prepare and cook them according to the directions and refrigerate in an airtight container up to 3 days. Reheat in the microwave or in a skillet and serve as directed.

variation: Substitute 2¼ cups cooked brown rice for the farro. This version is gluten-free (provided that you use gluten-free oats, bun, bread crumbs, and other ingredients).

PER SERVING: 354 calories, 11 g protein, 50 g carbohydrate, 15 g fat, 2 g saturated fat, 11 g fiber, 6 g sugar, 378 mg sodium
STAR NUTRIENTS: folate (18% DV), niacin (19% DV), pantothenic acid (11% DV), riboflavin (14% DV), thiamin (30% DV), vitamin A (53% DV), vitamin B6 (17% DV), vitamin C (17% DV), vitamin K (27% DV), copper (19% DV), iron (16% DV), magnesium (26% DV), manganese (84% DV), phosphorus (26% DV), potassium (18% DV), selenium (52% DV), zinc (17% DV)

steel-cut oats risotto with asparagus

ACTIVE PREPARATION TIME: **19 minutes** • TOTAL PREPARATION TIME: **31 minutes**

On a trip to Italy, I tasted a walnut risotto that was out of this world. Once I got home, I learned that you can make a risotto out of just about any whole grain in your pantry—even steel-cut oats. This whole grain boasts a lineup of wholesome nutrients, such as iron and magnesium. But the beta-glucan, a special fiber found in oats, is the real star of the nutrition party: just one daily serving has been linked with lowering blood cholesterol by up to 23 percent. Paired with savory flavors, almonds, and asparagus, this is a delicious way to get your daily oats!

MAKES 4 SERVINGS
(about 1¼ cups each)

1 tablespoon extra virgin olive oil
½ large onion, diced
2 medium garlic cloves, minced
1½ cups (105 g) sliced white mushrooms
½ teaspoon freshly ground black pepper
3 cups (711 ml) reduced sodium vegetable broth (see page 346)
½ cup (119 ml) white wine
1 cup (176 g) uncooked steel-cut oats
One 12-ounce (340 g) bunch fresh asparagus, ends trimmed,
    chopped into 1½-inch pieces
¼ cup (23 g) toasted sliced almonds
2 tablespoons chopped fresh sage, or 1 teaspoon dried

1. Heat the olive oil in a large saucepan over medium heat. Add the onions and sauté for 3 minutes.

2. Add the garlic, mushrooms, and black pepper and sauté for an additional 1 minute.

3. Meanwhile, heat the broth and wine in a small saucepan over medium heat until warm but not boiling.

4. Stir the oats into the vegetable mixture. Ladle approximately ½ cup of the warm broth mixture over it. Cook, uncovered, over medium heat, stirring frequently, until the liquid is absorbed. Repeat, adding ½ cup of the broth mixture at a time, as it is absorbed, cooking and stirring for 5 minutes. Add the asparagus, almonds, and sage, and continue cooking and adding more of the broth mixture until all the liquid has been incorporated and the risotto is creamy and just tender (15 to 20 additional minutes).

variation: Stir in one 15-ounce (425 g) can of drained beans (e.g., chickpeas, kidney, white, or fava) during step 4.

PER SERVING: 275 calories, 13 g protein, 37 g carbohydrate, 9 g fat, 1 g saturated fat, 8 g fiber, 4 g sugar, 52 mg sodium

STAR NUTRIENTS: folate (15% DV), niacin (16% DV), pantothenic acid (15% DV), riboflavin (25% DV), thiamin (13% DV), vitamin A (14% DV), vitamin B6 (11% DV), vitamin C (14% DV), vitamin E (12% DV), vitamin K (69% DV), calcium (10% DV), copper (33% DV), iron (25% DV), magnesium (10% DV), manganese (112% DV), molybdenum (13% DV), phosphorus (11% DV), potassium (13% DV), selenium (15% DV)

Miso-Braised Collard Greens with Cashews

Aim for at least six servings of veggies every day.

Miso-Braised Collard Greens with Cashews
Spaghetti Squash with Pomodoro Sauce and Pine Nuts
Jicama-Chayote Slaw

The world of vegetables offers an astonishing array. There are literally thousands of vegetables, in every shade of the rainbow and in all different shapes and sizes, from pearl-size green peas to swollen pumpkins the size of a child. And the flavors and textures are equally diverse. Just compare the sweet, smooth flesh of yams to the hot, crisp taste of habanero chiles!

Each vegetable is a nutrition powerhouse, offering you protein, fiber, and dozens of essential vitamins, minerals, and phytochemicals in each bite—and all for a skinny little calorie package. On average, vegetables provide about 25 calories, 2 grams of protein, and 5 grams of carbohydrates in a half-cup cooked serving. (Starchy veggies, like corn, potatoes, green peas, and winter squash have a bit more calories and carbs—though these are healthful choices, too—and dried beans and lentils fall under the category of legume, not veggie.) Studies show that people who feast on lots of vegetables reap rewards such as lower risks of certain cancers, type 2 diabetes, heart disease, cognitive decline, eye disease, and bone loss.

Yet, we fall short on our vegetable intake in this country. Many people don't even bite into their first vegetable serving until dinner (no, that parsley garnish or the slice of tomato on your sandwich doesn't count as a serving!), and then may be satisfied with one small portion. In order to gain the benefits of a whole foods, plant-based diet, I recommend that you aim for at least six daily servings of vegetables (generally 1 cup raw, ½ cup cooked).

It may seem easy, but it means you need to fit vegetables into nearly every meal and snack. Include them at breakfast, in a veggie breakfast burrito or sautéed with whole wheat toast. Pack carrot and celery sticks, broccoli and cauliflower florets, or snow peas for snacks. And double—or even triple—up on them at dinnertime by serving a one-dish vegetable stew, or adding a soup and salad. Don't be afraid to "sneak" vegetables into dishes, such as grated zucchini in taco filling and shredded carrots in cupcakes (see Carrot

Spice Cupcakes with Chocolate "Cream Cheese" Frosting, page 332). And if you've never been fond of vegetables, take a new venture into this plant world. Gone are the days of microwaved, bland, rubbery vegetables; they have been replaced with flavorful preparations, such as roasted (see Roasted Lemon-Sage Brussels Sprouts with Hazelnuts, page 62), sautéed in garlic and olive oil, or braised in miso (see Miso-Braised Collard Greens with Cashews, page 43). Make vegetables the *star* of your meal.

miso-braised collard greens with cashews

See photo on page 40

Some of the most nutritionally potent vegetables are deep-green leafy vegetables, such as collard greens. Here, they are combined with miso, a traditional Japanese paste made from fermented soy, for an easy dish with rich, savory taste. You may be familiar with miso from such iconic Japanese dishes as miso soup, but its umami flavoring complements many dishes. This simple braised green dish can be whipped up in minutes; alongside Easy Peanut Soba Noodles with Seitan (page 50), it becomes a delicious meal in less than half an hour.

MAKES 4 SERVINGS
(about 1 cup each)

1 teaspoon peanut oil
1 tablespoon miso paste (see Note)
⅓ cup (79 ml) water
Juice of ½ lemon
One 10-ounce (284 g) bunch collard greens, cleaned, trimmed, and coarsely chopped
¼ cup (35 g) raw cashews
1 tablespoon sliced dried seaweed

1. Combine the peanut oil, miso paste, water, and lemon juice in a large skillet over medium heat. Stir with a whisk until smooth and bubbly, about 2 minutes.

2. Add the collard greens, cover, and cook for about 4 minutes (without stirring), until the collards are barely tender but firm and bright green.

3. Garnish with the cashews and seaweed. Serve immediately.

note: Miso paste is available in many supermarkets, gourmet stores, and Asian markets. If following a gluten-free diet, use gluten-free miso paste and soy sauce.

variation: Add 6 ounces (170 g) sliced firm tofu (pressed, for best results— see page 103), tempeh, or seitan in step 2.

> **PER SERVING:** 119 calories, 5 g protein, 10 g carbohydrate, 8 g fat, 1 g saturated fat, 3 g fiber, 2 g sugar, 200 mg sodium
>
> **STAR NUTRIENTS:** folate (15% DV), vitamin A (48% DV), vitamin C (22% DV), vitamin K (230% DV), calcium (12% DV), iron (12% DV), magnesium (17% DV), phosphorus (11% DV)

spaghetti squash with pomodoro sauce and pine nuts

ACTIVE PREPARATION TIME: **20 minutes** • TOTAL PREPARATION TIME: **37 minutes**

Find unusual ways to get more veggies on your plate, such as starring veg-etables, like spaghetti squash, in a "pasta" dish. It's easy to understand where spaghetti squash gets its name—just cook it and watch its golden flesh turn into spaghetti-like strands. I paired this earthy squash "pasta" with a Pomodoro sauce—a simple, classic Italian tomato sauce—and crunchy toasted pine nuts. It's a surprisingly easy dish, yet so beautiful that it will look like you fussed over it for hours! Serve it with a side of sim-mered beans, such as Sicilian-Style Eye of the Goat Beans (page 96).

MAKES 8 SERVINGS
(one-eighth squash each)

1 medium spaghetti squash (about 4 pounds or 1,800 g)
1 tablespoon extra virgin olive oil
¼ medium onion, finely diced
3 medium garlic cloves, minced
One 28-ounce (794 g) can diced or crushed tomatoes, with
    liquid
¼ teaspoon smoked paprika
½ cup (20 g) chopped fresh basil leaves, or 1½ teaspoons dried
Pinch of freshly ground black pepper and/or sea salt, optional
3 tablespoons toasted pine nuts

1. Bring a large pot of water to boil.
2. Slice the squash in half horizontally and scoop out the seeds. Slice each half into 4 equal pieces, for a total of 8 pieces.
3. Add the squash to the boiling water, cover, and cook for about 20 min-utes on medium heat, until the squash is just tender, while not overcooked and soggy, and can be torn easily into strands with a fork. Drain off the water and cover the pot until serving time.
4. While the squash is cooking, heat the olive oil in a large skillet or sauté pan over medium heat.
5. Add the onion and sauté for about 4 minutes. Add the garlic and sauté an additional 4 minutes, until soft.
6. Add the onion mixture and tomatoes with their liquid to a blender and pulse for 2 to 3 seconds, just until well combined, yet still lumpy. Alter-natively, add the tomatoes and liquid to the onions and blend to the same texture using an immersion blender.

7. Return the tomato-onion mixture to the pan, add the paprika and basil, and heat until bubbly. Add the black pepper and sea salt, if desired.

8. To serve, place one wedge of spaghetti squash on each dinner plate. Loosen the strands with a fork. Spoon about ⅓ cup of sauce over each wedge and sprinkle with a heaping teaspoon of pine nuts. Serve immediately.

variations: Stir 10 ounces (283 g) of cubed baked tofu or sliced seitan into the sauce during step 7.

PER SERVING: 130 calories, 3 g protein, 22 g carbohydrate, 5 g fat, 1 g saturated fat, 5 g fiber, 9 g sugar, 78 mg sodium

STAR NUTRIENTS: niacin (12% DV), vitamin A (16% DV), vitamin B6 (13% DV), vitamin C (30% DV), vitamin K (16% DV), manganese (23% DV), phosphorus (16% DV), potassium (14% DV)

jicama-chayote slaw

ACTIVE PREPARATION TIME: **28 minutes** • TOTAL PREPARATION TIME: **28 minutes**

Crisp matchsticks of jicama and chayote—both plants native to Mexico—meld with grapefruit, avocado, chile, and limes to produce a cool, refreshing salad for the hottest of summer days. You can find jicama (the root of a vine) and chayote (a plant in the cucumber family) at most Latin supermarkets, and maybe even your nearby farmers market. I love serving this zesty salad to complement veggie taco night (see Tofu Mushroom Tacos on page 8) or grilled veggie burgers on a sunny afternoon.

MAKES 12 SERVINGS
(about 1 cup each)

1 medium jicama, sliced into thin matchsticks (510 g, about 4 cups)
One 9-ounce (255 g) chayote, sliced into thin matchsticks (see Note)
¼ medium red onion, thinly sliced
1 large pink grapefruit, peeled, segmented, chopped
1 medium avocado, chopped
1 cup (60 g) chopped fresh cilantro
1 small chile pepper (e.g., jalapeño, serrano, or habanero), finely diced
2 medium limes
2 tablespoons extra virgin olive oil
2 teaspoons agave nectar
2 cloves garlic, minced
½ teaspoon white pepper
Pinch of sea salt, optional

1. Mix together the jicama, chayote, onion, grapefruit, avocado, cilantro, and chile pepper in a large bowl.

2. Zest one lime into a small dish. Juice both limes and add to the dish, along with the olive oil, agave, garlic, white pepper, and sea salt, if desired. Whisk together.

3. Pour the dressing over the salad and toss together.

note: Chayote is available at many Latin markets, as well as the farmers market in some regions. If you can't find it, substitute 1 medium cucumber.

variations: You may substitute 2 medium oranges for the grapefruit.

PER SERVING: 83 calories, 1 g protein, 10 g carbohydrate, 5 g fat, 1 g saturated fat, 4 g fiber, 4 g sugar, 4 mg sodium
STAR NUTRIENTS: folate (10% DV), vitamin C (44% DV), vitamin K (12% DV)

Easy Peanut Soba
Noodles with Seitan

Read it before you eat it.

Easy Peanut Soba Noodles with Seitan
Zucchini-Orzo Soup
Bell Pepper Rye Pilaf

Most of your food purchases should be simple, minimally processed whole plant foods: whole grains such as oats and quinoa, legumes such as kidney beans and lentils, fresh fruits and vegetables, and nuts and seeds such as walnuts and sunflower seeds. Most of these foods don't come with complicated food labels, since they are single-ingredient foods. However, there's nothing wrong with relying on a few packaged foods, such as breakfast cereals, prepared breads, side dish mixes, and canned or frozen products to see you through. The good news is that many of these products boast a new dedication to whole plant foods—you can find pouches of pre-cooked ancient grains, canned unsalted beans, and hummus. But not all food products are created equal.

In your search for an optimal, whole plant foods diet, be picky about the products you purchase. The only way to achieve this is to read. Study two things on every food product label: the nutrition facts panel and the ingredients list. The nutrition facts will tell you the suggested serving size and the amount of calories, fat, saturated fat, protein, fiber, carbohydrates, and sodium in each. You want to keep your saturated fat and sodium levels down, and calories are of concern, too, if you're watching your weight. Look for products that contain 20% DV (Daily Value, based on 2,000 calories per day) or lower. In return, you want to see at least 10% DV of valuable nutrients, such as fiber and protein.

In many respects, the ingredients list is even more valuable. The first item listed has the greatest amount by weight, so it's a bad sign if it is oil, sugar, or refined grains, such as wheat flour or white rice. Instead, look for lots of whole plant foods and few artificial and refined ingredients. Make sure your hummus, for example, contains a fair amount of protein (3 g per serving is a nice contribution), not too much sodium (below 150 mg), and, most important, *real* ingredients.

See photo
on page 48

easy peanut soba noodles with seitan

ACTIVE PREPARATION TIME: **16 minutes** • TOTAL PREPARATION TIME: **16 minutes**

Who needs highly processed Asian noodle mixes when you can whip up this economical, family-size noodle dish in minutes? Paired with a crisp salad, such as the Spring Vegetable Salad with Green Goddess Dressing (page 000), it's a great solution for a busy weeknight dinner or quick Saturday lunch. Pack away the leftovers for lunch the next day—they'll be delicious served hot or cold.

MAKES 6 SERVINGS
(about 1 cup each)

3 cups (711 ml) water
One 7-ounce (198 g) package dried soba noodles
1 teaspoon sesame oil
1 medium bell pepper (red, yellow, or orange), coarsely chopped
1 cup (91 g) chopped broccoli
1 medium garlic clove, minced
1 teaspoon minced fresh ginger
½ teaspoon crushed red pepper
1 tablespoon chopped fresh basil, or 1 teaspoon dried
1 teaspoon sesame seeds (black or beige)
One 8-ounce (227 g) package plain seitan, sliced, drained
1 tablespoon unsalted creamy peanut butter
¼ cup (59 ml) reduced sodium vegetable broth (see page 346)
¼ cup (59 ml) orange juice
1½ tablespoons reduced sodium soy sauce
3 tablespoons coarsely chopped roasted peanuts
3 green onions, white and green parts, sliced

1. Place the water in a pot over high heat, cover, and bring to a boil. Add the soba, cover, and reduce heat to medium. Cook for about 5 minutes, until tender but firm. Place the noodles in a strainer and rinse.

2. While the noodles are cooking, heat the sesame oil in a large skillet over medium heat. Add the bell pepper, broccoli, garlic, ginger, crushed red pepper, basil, sesame seeds, and seitan. Sauté for 6 minutes.

3. Stir in the peanut butter, broth, juice, and soy sauce and cook, stirring, for 2 minutes.

4. Add the cooked, drained noodles and peanuts and sauté for about 2 minutes, until noodles are heated through.

5. Sprinkle with green onions and serve immediately.

variation: Substitute diced extra firm tofu (pressed, for best results—see page 103) for the seitan and/or rice noodles for the soba. (Using tofu and rice noodles makes the recipe gluten-free, provided that you check all other ingredients, such as the soy sauce, are gluten-free.)

PER SERVING: 221 calories, 11 g protein, 30 g carbohydrate, 7 g fat, .5 g saturated fat, 4 g fiber, 3 g sugar, 391 mg sodium
STAR NUTRIENTS: vitamin A (22% DV), vitamin C (68% DV), vitamin K (10% DV), calcium (10% DV), iron (13% DV), manganese (12% DV)

zucchini-orzo soup

ACTIVE PREPARATION TIME: **12 minutes** • TOTAL PREPARATION TIME: **50 minutes**

*Homemade, vegetable-based soups are one of the most nutritious, eco-
nomical, and easy things you can prepare. Chances are you'll have a
much lighter sodium load in a homemade version compared with many
canned soups, which can contain up to 1,600 milligrams per serving! In
the cooler months, let a pot of this soup simmer away while you prepare
the rest of your meal.*

MAKES 8 SERVINGS
(generous 1 cup each)

One 14.5-ounce (411 g) can diced tomatoes, no salt added, with
   liquid
6 cups (948 ml) water
2 teaspoons reduced sodium vegetable broth base
1 small onion, chopped
2 medium carrots, sliced
3 celery stalks, sliced
2 medium garlic cloves, minced
¼ teaspoon freshly ground black pepper
1 teaspoon dried basil
1 teaspoon dried oregano
Pinch of sea salt, optional
1 cup (180 g) dried whole grain orzo
2 small zucchinis, sliced

1. Add the tomatoes and water to a large pot and place it over medium-
high heat. Add the broth base, onion, carrots, celery, garlic, black pepper,
basil, and oregano.

2. Stir, cover, and bring to a simmer, then reduce the heat to medium and
cook for 25 minutes.

3. Taste and add a pinch of sea salt, if desired. Add the orzo and zucchini,
cover, and cook for an additional 15 minutes, until the vegetables are tender. You may need to add more water to replace moisture lost to evaporation, but the consistency should be thick.

note: This soup does not store well, because the orzo soaks up the liquid
in the soup during storage. If you don't plan on using the whole batch at
once, cut the recipe in half or freeze the extra portion immediately after
preparation.

variations: Substitute a yellow summer squash (or the leftover pulp from a stuffed squash recipe such as Yellow Squash Stuffed with Saffron Rye Berries, page 156) for one of the zucchinis. You could also try sprinkling a bit of za'atar on each bowl to brighten the flavors with Middle Eastern flair. (See page 345 to make your own.)

PER SERVING: 143 calories, 5 g protein, 29 g carbohydrate, 1 g fat, 0 g saturated fat, 6 g fiber, 6 g sugar, 63 mg sodium
STAR NUTRIENTS: folate (34% DV), niacin (13% DV), riboflavin (12% DV), thiamin (20% DV), vitamin A (68% DV), vitamin C (28% DV), iron (12% DV), potassium (10% DV)

bell pepper rye pilaf

ACTIVE PREPARATION TIME: **11 minutes** • TOTAL PREPARATION TIME: **1 hour**

Pilaf is a traditional savory grain dish that has a long history in many ethnic food cultures, including Greek, Persian, Turkish, and Indian. We have come to think of it as a packaged side dish that you can whip up in minutes. But you don't need a salty, highly processed box to put a delicious pilaf on the table. This Indian-inspired side dish relies on the nutty goodness of rye berries for a change of pace.

MAKES 8 SERVINGS
(about ¾ cup each)

1 tablespoon extra virgin olive oil
1 medium red onion, diced
1 teaspoon coriander
¼ teaspoon cayenne pepper
¼ teaspoon turmeric
1 teaspoon cumin seeds
1 teaspoon minced fresh ginger
2 medium garlic cloves, minced
1 medium red bell pepper, diced
1 medium yellow bell pepper, diced
2 cups (338 g) dried rye berries (see Notes)
4 cups (948 ml) water
1 tablespoon lemon juice
Pinch of sea salt, optional

1. Heat the olive oil in a large skillet or sauté pan over medium heat. Add the onion and sauté for 4 minutes. Add the coriander, cayenne, turmeric, cumin seeds, ginger, and garlic and sauté for an additional 4 minutes.

2. Add the red and yellow bell peppers and rye berries and continue to sauté for 4 minutes.

3. Add the water and lemon juice and cover the pan. Simmer on low heat for 45 to 50 minutes, stirring occasionally, until the rye berries are tender and the liquid is absorbed. Taste and add sea salt, if desired.

notes: You can find rye berries in most natural food stores and online whole grain purveyors.

If you prefer rice or follow a gluten-free diet, substitute 2 cups (285 g) brown rice in step 2, and 3 cups (710 ml) water in step 3, and cook until tender.

PER SERVING: 186 calories, 7 g protein, 38 g carbohydrate, 3 g fat, 0 g saturated fat, 7 g fiber, 2 g sugar, 6 mg sodium
STAR NUTRIENTS: vitamin A (19% DV), vitamin C (146% DV), iron (13% DV), phosphorus (20% DV)

Endive Salad with
Peas, Pea Shoots,
and Creamy
Lemon Dressing

9

Eat more, weigh less.

Pineapple and Mango with Coconut
Endive Salad with Peas, Pea Shoots, and Creamy Lemon Dressing
Roasted Lemon-Sage Brussels Sprouts with Hazelnuts

Weight loss is a mysterious thing. People spend $20 billion every year trying to lose weight. Research has, however, shown that a plant-based diet may be linked with a healthier weight. One new study found that the more plant-powered their diet, the less people weigh: vegans had on average a 5-point lower BMI than nonvegetarians (23.6 versus 28.8).

It makes sense, as most whole plant foods are *low-energy dense*, which means that they contain a relatively small amount of calories for the amount of food you get. For example, an ounce of cooked beef (85 percent lean) contains 70 calories, but an ounce of low-energy dense cooked spinach contains just 6 calories. Even plant foods that are slightly more energy dense, such as grains, beans, potatoes, and fruit, are relative calorie bargains. Cooked oats, for example, contain 154 calories per half-cup serving, and cooked pinto beans have 123 calories per one-half cup. These are nutrient bargains, compared to energy-dense foods like a Pizza Hut Meat Lover's pizza (350 calories per slice) or a half rack of baby back ribs (670 calories, with no sides).

Studies show that eating a diet rich in such low-energy, high-volume plant foods can be an effective weight loss strategy, thanks to their high fiber and water content, which fill you up for fewer calories. Case in point: you can enjoy a generous portion of stew that includes one-half cup each of quinoa, chickpeas, and mushrooms, plus one cup of green beans—and a half-cup serving of fresh strawberries for dessert—all for only 315 calories. That's the same amount of calories found in a fast-food kids' cheeseburger (not including toppings or fries!). Which meal would make you feel more content for longer? It's no wonder plant-powered eaters tend to consume fewer calories, and weigh less, than their meat-centric counterparts.

If you're trying to maintain or lose weight, load your plate with more of these nutrient-rich calorie bargains. Start your meal with a vegetable-rich soup or salad; fill your plate with vegetables; enjoy a fiber-rich whole grain and legume entrée, and feast on fruit for dessert. Don't count calories; count on whole plant foods.

pineapple and mango with coconut

ACTIVE PREPARATION TIME: **12 minutes** • TOTAL PREPARATION TIME: **12 minutes**

Fruits, which come in an array of colors, sizes, textures, and tastes, are perfect for eating just as they are. From inky purple blackberries to sunny oranges to showy dragon fruit, who needs dessert when you can bite into intoxicatingly perfumed, sweet fruits? In the tropical regions of Central America, the fresh fruit availability is almost obscene! You can observe bananas, coconuts, papayas, pineapples, mangoes, and more growing in the jungle—and for sale at local fruit stands. These fruits, which have grown in this region for centuries, are packed with flavor and nutrients. You can find such tropical fruits as I feature in this recipe in most super-markets today.

MAKES 12 SERVINGS
(about ¾ cup each)

2 tablespoons pine nuts
¼ cup (23 g) unsweetened shredded coconut
1 medium ripe pineapple, peeled, cored, and cut into 1½-inch
   chunks (see Note)
1 large ripe mango, peeled, cored, and cut into 1½-inch chunks
   (see Note)
1 medium banana, peeled and sliced
6 ounces (170 g or about ¾ cup) vanilla-flavored cultured coconut yogurt
2 tablespoons mango or orange juice

1. Preheat the oven or toaster oven to 375°F (190°C). Place the pine nuts and coconut in a shallow dish and bake for about 4 minutes, until browned (be careful not to burn). Remove from the oven and set aside to cool.

2. Place the pineapple, mango, and banana in a large mixing bowl.

3. In a small dish, combine the yogurt and mango or orange juice.

4. Fold the yogurt sauce into the fruit and coat well.

5. Sprinkle the toasted pine nuts and coconut onto the fruit and serve immediately.

note: Substitute canned pineapple chunks for fresh pineapple and frozen mango for fresh mango if unavailable or not in season.

PER SERVING: 86 calories, 1 g protein, 19 g carbohydrate, 1.5 g fat, 1 g saturated fat, 2 g fiber, 14 g sugar, 4 mg sodium
STAR NUTRIENTS: vitamin C (74% DV), vitamin E (11% DV), manganese (40% DV)

---

endive salad with peas, pea shoots, and creamy lemon dressing

ACTIVE PREPARATION TIME: **10 minutes** • TOTAL PREPARATION TIME: **10 minutes**

In order to find or maintain a healthy weight, start each meal with a salad—research shows it can help you eat less overall. Pea shoots—the tender tendrils of traditional pea plants—are becoming more and more popular among chefs and foodies alike. In this recipe, I layer their grassy pea flavor with green peas and a creamy lemony dressing. Piled on crisp endive leaves and garnished with chopped macadamia nuts, this salad is a stunner. It's the perfect accompaniment for a special meal, yet it looks much more difficult to make than it really is! This combination offers protein, fiber, vitamin C, and much more.

MAKES 4 SERVINGS
(1 salad each)

3 tablespoons reduced fat plant-based mayonnaise
(see page 343)
1 tablespoon lemon juice
1 teaspoon lemon zest
¼ teaspoon freshly ground black pepper
1 cup (134 g) frozen peas, thawed and drained (or fresh peas,
steamed and drained; see Notes)
2 Belgian endives, cleaned, trimmed, and cut in half horizontally
2 ounces (57 g) fresh pea shoots, ends trimmed (see Notes)
2 tablespoons chopped macadamia nuts

1. In a small dish, stir together the plant-based mayonnaise, lemon juice and zest, and black pepper. Fold in the peas.

2. Place the endive halves, cut side up, on 4 individual salad plates or one large platter.

3. Top each endive half with ¼ of the pea shoots (about ½ ounce) and ¼ cup of the pea mixture.

4. Sprinkle ½ tablespoon of the macadamia nuts onto each salad.

notes: You may substitute cooked shelled edamame, chickpeas, or beans (e.g., white beans, kidney beans, or black beans) for the peas.

If you can't find fresh pea shoots, substitute micro-sprouts or alfalfa sprouts.

PER SERVING: 125 calories, 5 g protein, 19 g carbohydrate, 5 g fat, 1 g saturated fat, 10 g fiber, 3 g sugar, 139 mg sodium
STAR NUTRIENTS: folate (28% DV), thiamin (20% DV), vitamin A (22% DV), vitamin C (32% DV), vitamin K (12% DV), magnesium (10% DV), manganese (28% DV), molybdenum (21% DV), phosphorus (10% DV), potassium (18% DV)

roasted lemon-sage brussels sprouts with hazelnuts

ACTIVE PREPARATION TIME: **7 minutes** • TOTAL PREPARATION TIME: **32 minutes**

Brussels sprouts are a great example of a low-energy, high-volume plant food. Chefs have fallen in love with these petite chou (tiny heads of cabbages). While these pungent buds got a bad name in the past—the only way most home cooks prepared brussels sprouts was to boil them to death—roasted brussels sprouts are all the rage today! Best of all, you can find this long-season, cold-loving vegetable fresh nearly year-round.

MAKES 4 SERVINGS
(about ½ cup each)

1 pound (454 g) fresh brussels sprouts, ends trimmed, halved
½ tablespoon extra virgin olive oil
1 tablespoon lemon juice
1 teaspoon roasted garlic, jarred or homemade (see Note)
1 teaspoon sliced fresh sage, or ½ teaspoon dried
Pinch of sea salt, optional
¼ cup (29 g) hazelnuts, coarsely chopped

1. Preheat the oven to 375°F (190°C).
2. Place the brussels sprouts in a casserole dish.
3. In a small dish, whisk together the olive oil, lemon juice, garlic, sage, and sea salt, if desired. Drizzle the oil mixture over the brussels sprouts and toss to coat.
4. Sprinkle the hazelnuts over the brussels sprouts.
5. Place in the oven on the top rack and roast for about 20 to 25 minutes, until brown and tender.

note: To make roasted garlic, trim the ends and papery outer covering of a whole bulb of garlic and place it in the center of a piece of foil in a small dish. Drizzle it with a teaspoon of olive oil, wrap it with the foil, and bake it at 375°F (180°C) for about 40 minutes, until browned and soft. Pop the cloves out of the bulb to serve or use as an ingredient.

variation: Add 8 ounces (227 g) of cubed extra firm tofu (pressed, for best results—see page 103) or sliced seitan during step 2.

PER SERVING: 112 calories, 5 g protein, 12 g carbohydrate, 6 g fat, .5 g saturated fat, 5 g fiber, 3 g sugar, 29 mg sodium
STAR NUTRIENTS: folate (20% DV), thiamin (14% DV), vitamin A (17% DV), vitamin B6 (15% DV), vitamin C (164% DV), vitamin E (11% DV), vitamin K (251% DV), iron (11% DV), magnesium (10% DV), manganese (43% DV), phosphorus (10% DV), potassium (14% DV)

Orange Millet Scones

10

Embrace whole grains for flavor and health.

Ruby Winter Quinoa Salad
Persian Couscous with Apricots and Pistachios
Orange Millet Scones
❧

The anti-grain movement is alive and well today. Fueled by a rise in gluten-free eating, as well as a so-called evolutionary eating philosophy, many people are questioning the value of grains altogether. However, if you eat these plant foods in their whole form—as close to nature as possible—and in reasonable portions, grains are indeed health-promoting. In fact, hundreds of studies have found that people who eat diets rich in whole grains reap lots of rewards, including lower risk of strokes, type 2 diabetes, heart disease, obesity, asthma, colorectal cancer, high blood pressure, and gum disease.

The conversation should not be about ditching *grains*, but about ditching *refined carbs* (see page 129). The benefit of eating grains comes in when you eat the *entire* grain. When wheat is milled into white flour, the outer bran layer and inner germ are stripped away, leaving only the starchy endosperm center. The resulting silky white flour is easily digested and rapidly absorbed into the bloodstream, thus promoting spikes in blood glucose and insulin production. That's why our penchant for highly refined grains, such as white bread, cookies, and snack crackers, has led to health problems.

Whole grains, essentially seeds of grass, provide key ingredients that you need for everyday life. Whole grains not only boast unique fibers and slow-burning carbs that fuel your body with energy but also provide rich supplies of B vitamins, as well as most of the minerals that your body needs to function properly. They can even give you a significant boost of antioxidants and protein.

That's not to say that people with gluten sensitivities or celiac disease (the autoimmune condition that is treated by avoiding gluten) should go against medical advice and consume gluten-containing grains (all varieties of wheat, barley, rye, and their crossbreeds). But even if you're on a gluten-free diet by medical necessity, you should still gain the benefits of consuming wholesome gluten-free grains, such as buckwheat, brown rice, quinoa, and millet.

Steam whole grains in water as you would rice, and try adding whole grain wheat, quinoa, and amaranth flours in baking (if you're unsure, start by replacing a quarter of the white flour in a recipe with whole grain flour and gradually increase the amount as you get used to the taste and texture). Don't limit yourself to just one; try them all: amaranth, barley, brown rice, buckwheat, corn, millet, oats, quinoa, teff, whole wheat, wild rice and more.

ruby winter quinoa salad

ACTIVE PREPARATION TIME: **15 minutes** • TOTAL PREPARATION TIME: **25 minutes**

Let whole grains reign supreme at every meal, in cereal, breads, side dishes, and even salads. Simple ancient grains—such as quinoa, a fiber- and protein-rich diet staple in Peru—are excellent in salads, such as this winter recipe. When the cool weather comes, turn to fall and winter fruits, such as pomegranates and pears, to flavor a crunchy grain salad. The ruby fruits, grains, and lettuce in this salad paint it red—a calling card for powerful phytochemicals with disease-fighting potential. The salad itself is simple enough for a weeknight dinner yet elegant enough for your holiday table. It's delicious—and substantial—enough to pack up in a lunch box for the next day.

MAKES 6 SERVINGS
(generous 1 cup each)

2 cups (474 ml) water
1 cup (170 g) uncooked red (or multicolored) quinoa
½ teaspoon reduced sodium vegetable broth base
1 cup (113 g) fresh pomegranate arils (seeds)
¼ cup (40 g) finely chopped red onion
2 medium celery stalks, diced
1 medium red pear, with peel, cored and diced
¼ cup (35 g) sunflower seeds
2 tablespoons pomegranate molasses (see Notes on page 177)
½ tablespoon red wine vinegar
½ tablespoon extra virgin olive oil
2 tablespoons sunflower seed butter
¼ teaspoon freshly ground black pepper
2 tablespoons chopped fresh parsley, or 1 teaspoon dried
　　parsley flakes
½ teaspoon low-sodium herbal seasoning blend (see page 345)
1 medium garlic clove, minced
2 cups (72 g) loosely packed baby red leaf lettuce

1. Add the water to a small pot and bring to a boil over high heat, then add the quinoa and broth base and reduce the heat to medium. Cover and cook for 15 minutes (or follow the package directions, which may vary slightly). Transfer the quinoa to a bowl and chill until cool.

recipe continues

2. Meanwhile, combine the pomegranate arils, onion, celery, pear, and sunflower seeds in a medium bowl.

3. In a small dish, make the dressing by stirring together the pomegranate molasses, vinegar, olive oil, sunflower seed butter, black pepper, parsley, herbal seasoning, and garlic until creamy.

4. Add the cooled quinoa to the pomegranate aril mixture and stir well. Add the dressing and toss well to coat.

5. Line a platter or salad bowl with the lettuce. Top with the quinoa salad. Serve immediately, or chill until serving time.

variations: Substitute 2 cups of cooked whole grains, such as sorghum, wheat berries, brown rice, or farro for the quinoa, or use 2 cups of any other variety of cooked quinoa, such as white (golden) or black.

PER SERVING: 234 calories, 8 g protein, 32 g carbohydrate, 9 g fat, 1 g saturated fat, 5 g fiber, 7 g sugar, 39 mg sodium

STAR NUTRIENTS: folate (17% DV), thiamin (11% DV), vitamin A (117% DV), vitamin C (14% DV), vitamin E (18% DV), vitamin K (168% DV), copper (13% DV), iron (19% DV), magnesium (12% DV), manganese (22% DV), phosphorus (11% DV), potassium (10% DV), selenium (14% DV)

persian couscous with apricots and pistachios

ACTIVE PREPARATION TIME: **11 minutes** • TOTAL PREPARATION TIME: **31 minutes**

The spices and flavors—ginger, cardamom, turmeric, pistachios—of the Middle East are abundant in this fragrant side dish, which features couscous, the traditional wheat-based food of North Africa. By dipping into such aromatic and flavorful herbs and spices, you can power up the appeal of foods without the aid of salt. Serve this couscous with a legume recipe, such as Chickpea Stew with Kale and Za'atar (page 12), for a punch of whole grain goodness, heart-healthy fiber intake, and anti-inflammatory spice power.

MAKES 6 SERVINGS
(about ¾ cup each)

½ tablespoon extra virgin olive oil
1 medium onion, diced
½ teaspoon minced fresh ginger
¼ teaspoon cardamom
¼ teaspoon cinnamon
¼ teaspoon turmeric
Pinch of cayenne pepper (see Notes)
½ cup (60 g) chopped dried apricots
1½ cups (171 g) pearled (Israeli) whole wheat couscous (see Notes)
2½ cups (593 ml) reduced sodium vegetable broth (see page 000)
⅓ cup (41 g) shelled pistachios

1. Heat the olive oil in a large saucepan over medium heat. Add the onion and cook for 4 minutes. Add the ginger, cardamom, cinnamon, turmeric, and cayenne and cook for an additional 4 minutes, stirring frequently.
2. Add the apricots, couscous, and broth. Stir well and cover. Reduce the heat to medium-low and simmer for about 20 minutes, stirring frequently to avoid sticking, until the couscous is tender and the liquid is absorbed.
3. Sprinkle with the pistachios and serve.

notes: Omit or slightly increase the amount of cayenne to adjust for your desired spice preference.

Pearled (or Israeli) whole wheat couscous, available in natural food and specialty stores, is a larger variety and takes longer to cook than the traditional couscous.

recipe continues

variation: To make this gluten-free, substitute brown rice couscous, adding more broth as needed in step 2; cooking time should be reduced by about 5 minutes. Check that all other ingredients are gluten-free.

PER SERVING: 282 calories, 10 g protein, 51 g carbohydrate, 6 g fat, .5 g saturated fat, 8 g fiber, 10 g sugar, 38 mg sodium
STAR NUTRIENTS: iron (12% DV)

orange millet scones

See photo
on page 64

ACTIVE PREPARATION TIME: **11 minutes** • TOTAL PREPARATION TIME: **36 minutes**

*These tender scones are full of zesty orange flavor and a crunchy pop,
thanks to the millet kernels tucked into the dough—proof that whole grains
can mean much more than just whole wheat. The scones are layered with
both millet flour and whole millet, a longtime nutrient-dense staple of Africa, Asia, and India. I love to serve these fragrant breads as a snack with
coffee or as an accompaniment to a simple meal, such as Tofu Cobb Salad
(page 82).*

MAKES 6 SERVINGS
(1 large scone each)

Nonstick cooking spray
2 tablespoons chia seeds (see Notes)
1 tablespoon egg replacer (e.g., Ener-G; see Notes)
¼ cup (85 g) honey or agave nectar
¼ cup (59 ml) unsweetened plain plant-based milk
5 tablespoons soft dairy-free margarine (see Notes on page 223)
1½ teaspoons fresh orange zest
½ cup (60 g) millet flour (see Notes)
½ cup (60 g) whole wheat pastry flour
½ cup (100 g) uncooked whole millet
1 tablespoon baking powder

1. Preheat the oven to 375°F (190°C). Spray a baking sheet with nonstick
cooking spray.
2. Mix the chia seeds, egg replacer, honey, and plant-based milk together
with an electric mixer or vigorously with a whisk for 2 minutes.
3. Add the margarine and combine well.
4. Stir in the orange zest, millet flour, whole wheat pastry flour, whole
millet, and baking powder just until combined to make a soft dough (do not
overmix).
5. Drop the batter by large spoonfuls onto the prepared sheet to make 6
scones.
6. Bake for 20 minutes, until golden brown. Serve warm.

notes: Egg replacer (e.g., Ener-G), available at many natural food stores,
can replace eggs in many baked dishes. Made of various plant starches and

recipe continues

Embrace whole grains for flavor and health. • 71

gums, egg replacer creates a light fluffy texture in these scones. The chia seeds also offer emulsification properties in this recipe. Although the egg replacer produces the best results in this recipe, you can omit it and add 2 tablespoons of additional whole wheat flour.

Millet flour is available at many natural food stores and online. If you can't find it, you may replace it with an additional ½ cup of whole wheat pastry flour.

You may store leftovers in an airtight container at room temperature for a few days or freeze for up to one month.

variations: You can make mini-scones by dropping 12 smaller spoonfuls onto the baking sheet in step 5. You may also substitute lemon zest for the orange zest to make Lemon Millet Scones. To make this recipe gluten-free, substitute a gluten-free flour blend (such as Bob's Red Mill or King Arthur Flour) for the whole wheat pastry flour and confirm that all other ingredients are gluten-free.

PER SERVING: 262 calories, 6 g protein, 40 g carbohydrate, 9 g fat, 1 g saturated fat, 5 g fiber, 11 g sugar, 90 mg sodium
STAR NUTRIENTS: niacin (12% DV), thiamin (14% DV), vitamin C (11% DV), calcium (35% DV), iron (11% DV), magnesium (17% DV)

Good meals don't just happen— plan them wisely.

Sweet Potato Gnocchi with Pistachio-Orange Pesto

Tropical Red Cabbage and Spelt Salad

❦

It's easy to get excited about all of the benefits you, your family, and the planet will gain by eating a whole-foods, plant-powered diet. But like a newly planted fruit tree, this optimal style of eating won't develop unless you nurture it. If you start with a little careful planning first, you will soon be able to enjoy the fruits of your labor.

Follow these planning tips to create healthy, plant-powered meals every day:

- **Pick your best shopping days.** Strategize your shopping around your schedule. For example, if you work Monday through Friday, you may want to shop for staples on Saturday or Sunday. Check out your local farmers market or rely on the offerings from your CSA for fresh produce, and plan this into your shopping schedule as well (see page 99 for more on CSAs).

- **Plan your menu.** Before your shopping trip, it might be helpful to get out a pad of paper or your smartphone and write up a brief menu for the week. This is the basis for your shopping list.

- **Don't be afraid to plan meals on the fly.** If you're not a menu person, then make sure your refrigerator is full of the freshest, most delectable produce of the season—whether from your supermarket, farmers market, or CSA—and your shelves are full of pantry staples (see "Collect a plant-powered pantry arsenal," page 35). Then all you have to do is combine fresh produce with beans, whole grains, and seasonings to create delicious meals at the drop of a hat.

- **Write out a shopping list.** Whether you take a menu-writing or spur-of-the moment approach, you'll be much more efficient (and save last-minute shopping trips) if you write out a shopping list.

sweet potato gnocchi with pistachio-orange pesto

ACTIVE PREPARATION TIME: **30 minutes** • TOTAL PREPARATION TIME: **1 hour**

If you want to enjoy delicious, plant-powered meals, keep a supply of staples on hand, such as root vegetables, extra virgin olive oil, and nuts. You might be surprised to find out that homemade gnocchi—those classic Italian mini-dumplings—are quite simple to make. Just whip up your dough, roll it into ropes, slice the ropes into "pillows," and drop them into boiling water—no need for any special pasta-making equipment. You can even make it easier with a little planning, if you cook the sweet potatoes the day before. My sweet potato gnocchi is rich in flavor, color, and antioxidants, and pairs beautifully with this zesty orange pistachio pesto. Serve this dish with French Lentil Salad with Cherry Tomatoes (page 26) for a fresh, European take on gorgeous plant-powered cuisine.

MAKES 8 SERVINGS
(½ cup gnocchi and 1 tablespoon pesto)

Gnocchi
2 large (567 g) sweet potatoes, peeled and cubed (see Notes)
¼ teaspoon nutmeg
Pinch of kosher salt, optional
2 cups (240 g) white whole wheat flour, plus more for rolling
6 to 12 tablespoons unsweetened plain plant-based milk
1 teaspoon extra virgin olive oil

Pistachio-Orange Pesto
½ cup (62 g) toasted shelled unsalted pistachios
Juice of ½ lemon
2 tablespoons orange juice
Zest of ½ medium orange
1½ teaspoons extra virgin olive oil
Pinch of freshly ground black pepper

1. To make the gnocchi, place sweet potatoes in a small pot and cover with water. Cover and bring to a boil over high heat. Reduce the heat and simmer for about 20 minutes, until tender. Drain the sweet potatoes, place in a mixing bowl, and mash well with a potato masher. Cool slightly.

2. Meanwhile, prepare the pesto by combining all of the ingredients in a small food processor or blender. Process until smooth but chunky (do not overprocess), scraping down the sides if necessary. Set aside.

3. Mix the mashed sweet potatoes with the nutmeg, kosher salt (if desired), and flour with an electric mixer. Add enough plant-based milk, 1 tablespoon at a time, to make a soft, slightly sticky dough.

4. Turn out the dough onto a clean, floured surface and separate into 6 pieces. Roll each piece into a 1-inch rope, then cut into 1-inch segments to create "pillows."

5. Fill a large pot with several inches of water and bring to a boil, then reduce the heat to a simmer. Add the olive oil.

6. Add half of the pillows of gnocchi dough to the boiling water. Once they rise to the top, cook for an additional 5 to 8 minutes, until the gnocchi are cooked through. Remove with a slotted spoon and drain. Repeat to cook the next batch of gnocchi.

7. Serve immediately, with the pesto.

notes: You can use frozen, thawed sweet potatoes in step 3.

The Pistachio-Orange Pesto is also an excellent accompaniment to other pasta dishes, sandwiches, or vegetable sides. You can double this pesto recipe, which stores well in an airtight container in the refrigerator for up to one week.

Though the gnocchi is best enjoyed fresh, you can store leftovers in the refrigerator (separately from the pesto) for up to 3 days and reheat in the microwave later. You can also make up the gnocchi the day before and boil when you plan to eat it.

variation: To make this gluten-free, substitute an all-purpose gluten-free flour blend (such as Bob's Red Mill or King Arthur Flour) for the white whole wheat flour, and add enough plant-based milk (1 tablespoon at a time) to create a soft, slightly sticky dough.

PER SERVING: 191 calories, 6 g protein, 32 g carbohydrate, 6 g fat, 1 g saturated fat, 6 g fiber, 3 g sugar, 13 mg sodium
STAR NUTRIENTS: niacin (11% DV), thiamin (17% DV), vitamin A (125% DV), vitamin B6 (18% DV), vitamin C (24% DV), magnesium (15% DV), potassium (10% DV)

Tropical Red Cabbage
and Spelt Salad

tropical red cabbage and spelt salad

ACTIVE PREPARATION TIME: **15 minutes** • TOTAL PREPARATION TIME: **50 minutes**

Spelt, an ancient variety of wheat, offers a nutty crunch to salads. Combined with exotic dried fruits and spices, and colorful red cabbage, this salad can hold its own on the dinner table. Pair it with a bean or lentil stew, such as my Black Bean–Corn Chili (page 236) for a wholesome, satisfying plant-powered meal. And it will taste just as good packed away for a to-go lunch the next day.

MAKES 8 SERVINGS
(scant 1 cup each)

¾ cup (131 g) uncooked spelt (see Notes)
3 cups (711 ml) water
8 ounces (227 g) shredded red cabbage (about 4 cups; see Notes)
¾ cup (227 g) chopped dried tropical fruit (e.g., pineapple, papaya, mango)
3 green onions, white and green parts, sliced
½ cup (30 g) chopped fresh parsley
1 tablespoon hemp seeds
3 tablespoons orange juice
1 tablespoon extra virgin olive oil
1 medium garlic clove, minced
¼ teaspoon crushed red pepper
½ teaspoon ground cumin
½ teaspoon chili powder
¼ teaspoon turmeric

1. Place the spelt and water in a small pot. Cover and cook on medium heat for 45 to 50 minutes, stirring occasionally, until tender. Cool slightly.
2. Once cooled, toss together the spelt, red cabbage, dried fruit, green onions, parsley, and hemp seeds in a large bowl.
3. In a small bowl, make the dressing by whisking together the orange juice, olive oil, garlic, crushed red pepper, cumin, chili powder, and turmeric.
4. Add the dressing to the salad and toss.

notes: Make the spelt the night before to save time whipping up this recipe.
   You can find preshredded red cabbage in the produce section at most supermarkets.

recipe continues

variation: Substitute ¾ cup (147 g) brown basmati rice for the spelt in step 1, and cook with 1½ cups water for 40 minutes.

PER SERVING: 136 calories, 4 g protein, 24 g carbohydrate, 4 g fat, .5 g saturated fat, 4 g fiber, 8 g sugar, 16 mg sodium
STAR NUTRIENTS: vitamin A (25% DV), vitamin C (77% DV), magnesium (10% DV)

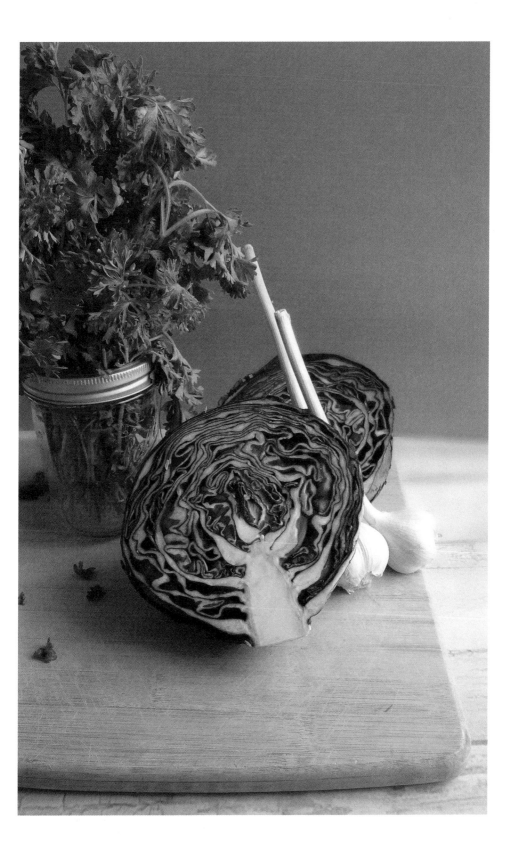

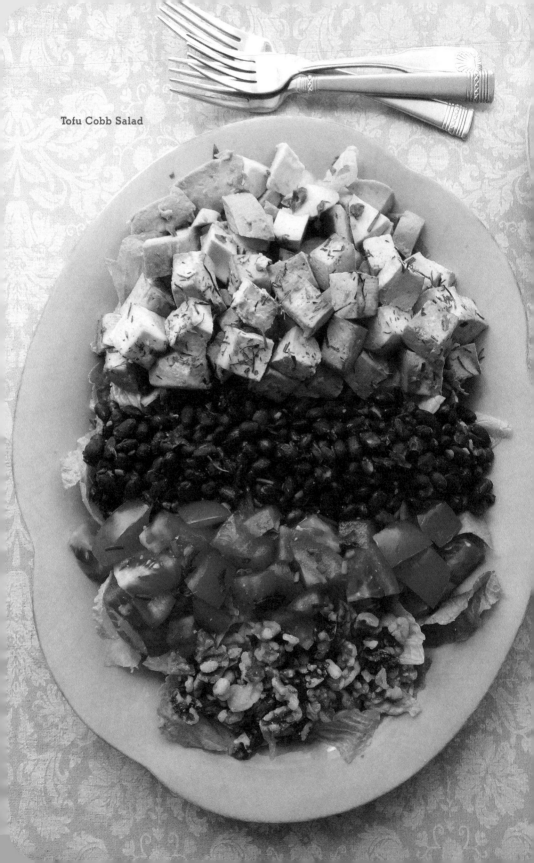

Tofu Cobb Salad

Make variety your motto.

Tofu Cobb Salad

Polenta with Puttanesca Sauce

Rosemary and Olive Cassoulet (Bean Stew)

We're creatures of habit, including in our food choices. Consumer research shows that people often eat the same thing every day for breakfast and choose the same foods in supermarkets on each shopping trip. How many times do you order your favorite lunch at your neighborhood restaurant, and pick up your favorite breakfast cereal in the supermarket? It's great to know your tastes, especially when you understand the nutritional value and background of your favorite foods. But variety should come first—your health depends upon it.

If you eat only iceberg lettuce and never the dark green leaves of arugula, kale, and spinach, you're missing out on a cache of vitamins, minerals, phytochemicals, and protein. If you eat potatoes as a side dish at every dinner, you're missing out on the nutrients and flavors found in brown rice, barley, and buckwheat. One plant may be rich in iron, while another may be rich in calcium. One plant may be potent in vitamin C, while another may pack B vitamins. Diversity at every meal, all day long, stokes your diet with a powerful combination of macro- and micronutrients that have important benefits for your body's organs and tissues. While it may be difficult to meet 100 percent of your needs for each nutrient every day, when you eat a wholesome diet with a great deal of variety, you can fill those little gaps over the course of your week.

So, don't get too stuck on the same things every day—mix it up! Try oats instead of toast for breakfast (see Scandinavian Apple-Cardamom Oatmeal, page 212) for a boost of beta-glucans—fiber linked with heart protection. Sprinkle chopped Brazil nuts onto your plant-based yogurt once in a while for a selenium surge. Try black beans one day (for a dose of brain-healthy anthocyanins) and pinto the next (for iron and calcium). Another side benefit of variety? A delicious, flavorful, colorful spectrum of tastes and textures. *Viva la différence!*

See photo
on page 80

tofu cobb salad

ACTIVE PREPARATION TIME: **15 minutes** • TOTAL PREPARATION TIME: **15 minutes**

Who says plant-powered eaters can't enjoy a Cobb salad now and again? Especially if you swap out a few of the animal foods in a classic Cobb for these plant superstars, including baked tofu and black beans. It's an easy, colorful entrée salad, which furnishes a rainbow of vibrant plant foods, including tomatoes, avocados, walnuts, and fresh herbs. Pair it with a whole grain vegetable soup, such as Zucchini-Orzo Soup (page 52).

MAKES 8 SERVINGS
(about 1¼ cups each)

....

6 cups (282 g) torn, loosely packed romaine lettuce
1 tablespoon extra virgin olive oil
1 teaspoon red wine vinegar
1 tablespoon finely minced fresh herbs (e.g., oregano, tarragon,
　　thyme), or ½ teaspoon dried
¼ teaspoon ground mustard
1 small garlic clove, minced
¼ teaspoon freshly ground black pepper
Pinch of sea salt, optional
1 cup (185 g) cooked black beans, no salt added, rinsed and
　　drained if canned
8 ounces (227 g) baked tofu (savory flavor), cubed (see Note)
2 small tomatoes, diced
1 medium avocado, peeled, cored, and diced
1 teaspoon lemon juice
½ cup (58 g) walnut pieces
2 tablespoons minced fresh chives

1. Place the lettuce in a mixing bowl.

2. Whisk together the olive oil, vinegar, herbs, mustard, garlic, black pepper, and sea salt, if desired, in a small dish. Add to the lettuce and toss well.

3. Place the dressed lettuce on an oval platter in a uniform layer.

4. Arrange the black beans on top of the lettuce, creating a row in the center of the platter.

5. To the right of the black beans, create a row of baked tofu.

6. To the left of the black beans, create a row of tomatoes.

7. Sprinkle the avocados with the lemon juice to avoid discoloration and arrange them in a narrower row to the right of the baked tofu.

8. To the left of the tomatoes, create a single smaller row of walnut pieces.

9. Sprinkle the entire salad with the chives.

10. Serve immediately.

note: Baked tofu is marinated, seasoned tofu, which is available in the refrigerator section in many supermarkets. It is an excellent addition to salads and sandwiches. You can make your own this way: Preheat the oven to 350°F (180°C). Slice 8 ounces of pressed tofu (see page 000) in half lengthwise into two rectangles. Place the rectangles into a small baking dish and drizzle with 2 tablespoons reduced sodium soy sauce and additional herbs and spices, as desired. Bake the tofu for 20 to 25 minutes.

variation: Substitute any colorful cooked bean for the black beans, such as cranberry beans, kidney beans, pink beans, or green flageolet beans.

PER SERVING: 195 calories, 11 g protein, 12 g carbohydrate, 13 g fat, 1.5 g saturated fat, 5 g fiber, 1 g sugar, 125 mg sodium
STAR NUTRIENTS: folate (23% DV), vitamin A (78% DV), vitamin C (13% DV), vitamin K (50%), copper (10% DV), iron (11% DV), manganese (23% DV), molybdenum (29% DV), potassium (10% DV)

polenta with puttanesca sauce

ACTIVE PREPARATION TIME: **15 minutes** • TOTAL PREPARATION TIME: **52 minutes**

*Don't stick with the same old side dish, such as rice or potatoes. Take
your appetite on a cultural adventure by sampling from a range of whole
grains. Polenta, based on cornmeal, started out as a humble European
staple made of ground wheat and other grains or chickpeas before corn's
arrival from the New World. Once corn was introduced to the Old World,
polenta evolved into a creamy cornmeal porridge, which was cooked up
in a copper pot and topped with flavorful sauces and toppings. In my
no-stir, plant-powered version, I pair polenta with another classic peasant
recipe—puttanesca sauce. Based on a few simple ingredients, such as tomatoes, capers, olives, onions, and garlic, it follows the timeworn tradition
of featuring only simple ingredients gleaned from the region—an Italian
trademark.*

MAKES 8 SERVINGS
(about 1 cup combined polenta and sauce each)

Polenta
1 cup (156 g) uncooked polenta (corn grits; see Notes)
3½ cups (830 ml) water
Pinch of kosher salt, optional
1 teaspoon extra virgin olive oil

Puttanesca Sauce
½ tablespoon extra virgin olive oil
1 medium onion, diced
3 medium garlic cloves, minced
One 28-ounce (794 g) can diced tomatoes, no salt added, with
    juice
1 tablespoon tomato paste
3 tablespoons capers, rinsed and drained
½ cup (64 g) packed Italian olives (e.g., Castelvetrano, Ceri-
    gnola, Bitetto), pitted and halved
½ teaspoon dried basil
½ teaspoon crushed red pepper

1. Preheat the oven to 350°F (180°C).
2. To make the polenta, pour the polenta, water, salt (if desired), and 1
teaspoon of olive oil into an 8-cup (1,896 ml) baking dish. Stir well. Bake
uncovered for 50 minutes.
3. Meanwhile, to make the Puttanesca Sauce, heat the olive oil in a pan
over medium heat. Add the onion and garlic and sauté for 6 minutes.

4. Add the tomatoes, tomato paste, capers, olives, basil, and crushed red pepper. Stir together and cook on low for 15 minutes, uncovered, stirring occasionally, until the sauce is thickened.

5. After 50 minutes, when the polenta is firm, remove it from the oven, pour the hot Puttanesca Sauce on top, and serve.

notes: Uncooked polenta, or corn grits, is essentially coarsely ground bits of corn (see page 247 for more information).

You may serve this dish with plant-based Parmesan "cheese" (such as Go Veggie! Parmesan Grated Topping), if desired. Alternatively, or in addition, add toasted pine nuts, pistachio nuts, or cooked white beans to the sauce in step 4.

PER SERVING: 166 calories, 4 g protein, 26 g carbohydrate, 5 g fat, 1 g saturated fat, 3 g fiber, 4 g sugar, 373 mg sodium
STAR NUTRIENTS: vitamin A (13% DV), vitamin C (30% DV)

rosemary and olive cassoulet (bean stew)

ACTIVE PREPARATION TIME: **10 minutes** • TOTAL PREPARATION TIME: **1 hour 35 minutes** (not including soaking time)

There's no need to get stuck in a rut on a plant-powered diet. Doing so would be not only bad for your palate but also bad for your health, because you miss out on the unique nutrient profiles found in each and every plant. Thousands of plant food varieties around the globe can inspire diverse, flavorful meals. Take these mint-green heirloom flageolet beans, which were a favorite of French chefs during the nineteenth century. Their earthy taste and creamy texture make flageolet beans a perfect match for French-Mediterranean cassoulets (bean stews), such as this dish. Search your natural food store or an online purveyor for this bean variety, or substitute a creamy white bean, such as great northern beans or lima beans.

MAKES 6 SERVINGS
(about ¾ cup each)

12 ounces (340 g, or about 2 cups) dried green flageolet beans
   or great northern or lima beans
4 cups (948 ml) water, plus more for soaking
½ tablespoon reduced sodium vegetable broth base
2 bay leaves
2 medium garlic cloves, minced
½ teaspoon freshly ground black pepper
½ tablespoon extra virgin olive oil
⅓ cup (43 g) drained olives (such as Sicilian or kalamata)
4 rosemary sprigs

1. Place the beans in a medium pot and cover with water. Cover and soak overnight.
2. Drain and rinse the beans and return them to the pot.
3. Add the water, broth base, bay leaves, garlic, and pepper, stirring well.
4. Cover and bring to a boil over high heat. Reduce the heat to medium and simmer for 45 minutes.
5. Remove the lid and cook for an additional 45 to 50 minutes, until the liquid is concentrated and beans are just tender but not bursting.
6. Drizzle the olive oil onto the beans and top with the olives and rosemary. Cover the pot and set it aside for 20 to 30 minutes to allow the flavors to mingle.

note: Steps 2 through 6 are perfectly suited for the slow cooker. Set it to high and cook for 4 to 5 hours.

PER SERVING: 237 calories, 14 g protein, 39 g carbohydrate, 3.5 g fat, .5 g saturated fat, 13 g fiber, 2 g sugar, 182 mg sodium

STAR NUTRIENTS: folate (74% DV), thiamin (27% DV), vitamin B6 (15% DV), calcium (12% DV), iron (20% DV), magnesium (30% DV), phosphorus (21% DV), potassium (25% DV), zinc (10% DV)

Mediterranean
Eggplant and
Artichoke Lasagna

Shop thoughtfully and purposefully.

Ethiopian Yam and Lentil Stew
Mediterranean Eggplant and Artichoke Lasagna
Sicilian-Style Eye of the Goat Beans

S o, you're organized, and you have your menu and your shopping list in hand, but it can all break down in the supermarket aisles if you can't find chia seeds and almond butter, or if you get bogged down choosing between products. It's no wonder that so many people find food shopping to be a dreaded chore.

Follow my steps to lighten your load and create smart food-shopping strategies to support your plant-powered eating style.

- **Pinpoint the best plant-powered supermarket in your community.** Do some scouting in your neighborhood and find the stores that best meet your plant-powered needs in your community. If time is a priority, try to avoid making multiple stops at several stores each week. Zero in on supermarkets that support the plant-powered life-style by stocking a variety of whole grains and legumes, a good selection of dried herbs and spices, a nice fresh produce section that focuses on local, seasonal produce, and an array of plant-based foods, such as milks, yogurts, tofu, seitan, and tempeh. And don't rule out the Internet, which is an increasingly useful way to purchase staples such as grains, nuts, and legumes.
- **Make thoughtful food purchases.** While it's important to read nutri-tion information before you make food choices (see "Read it before you eat it," page 49), it's also important to get to know what your favorite food companies are all about. You might want to consider doing a little homework on the computer (or even on your smart-phone in the aisles) by checking out their websites—do they have a focus on sustainability, giving back, and wellness? Support the best food companies with your shopping dollars.
- **Look beyond nutrition.** Good, healthy food is more than just a pack-age of carbohydrates, protein, and vitamins. As much as possible,

it should also be flavorful, low in pesticide residues (i.e., organic), local, and whole (see page 267).

◄ **Save dollars with good food.** You don't have to shop at a high-priced natural food store to eat a healthful plant-based diet. Remember, this eating style—low in animal proteins and highly processed foods—should *save* you money, not cost you more. Look for nutrition bargains: seasonal fresh fruit and bins of grains, legumes, nuts, and seeds.

ethiopian yam and lentil stew

ACTIVE PREPARATION TIME: **18 minutes** • TOTAL PREPARATION TIME: **1 hour**

Ethiopian cuisine represents some of the most flavorful plant-based food on the planet! That's thanks to ingredients like shelf-stable dried legumes, root vegetables, and exotic spices. Once you've got these ingredients on hand, this recipe is an easy one-dish meal solution, served with whole grain flatbread on the side.

MAKES 4 SERVINGS
(generous 1 cup each)

1½ teaspoons peanut oil
1 large onion, diced
3 medium garlic cloves, minced
1 teaspoon minced fresh ginger
1 large (283 g) fresh yam or sweet potato, diced
½ medium green bell pepper, diced
1 cup (192 g) dried red lentils
One 14.5-ounce (411 g) can diced tomatoes, no salt added, with
    liquid
4 cups (948 ml) water
½ teaspoon sweet paprika
¼ teaspoon cayenne pepper
1 teaspoon cumin
¼ teaspoon nutmeg
Pinch of ground cloves
½ teaspoon cinnamon
Pinch of kosher salt, optional
2 tablespoons lemon juice
¼ cup (15 g) chopped fresh parsley
¼ cup (10 g) chopped fresh mint

1. Heat the peanut oil in a large, heavy pot over medium heat. Add the onion and sauté for 5 minutes.

2. Add the garlic, ginger, yam, and bell pepper and sauté for an additional 5 minutes.

3. Add the lentils, tomatoes, water, paprika, cayenne, cumin, nutmeg, cloves, and cinnamon. Stir well, bring to a simmer, reduce the heat to medium-low, cover, and simmer for 35 to 40 minutes, until the lentils and vegetables are tender. Taste and add a pinch of kosher salt, if desired.

recipe continues

4. Add the lemon juice, parsley, and mint and stir well. Cover and simmer for an additional 5 minutes.

variation: Substitute one 15-ounce (425 g) can of drained chickpeas or red beans for the lentils in step 2 and cook until vegetables are tender.

PER SERVING: 166 calories, 10 g protein, 29 g carbohydrate, 2 g fat, 0 g saturated fat, 12 g fiber, 5 g sugar, 40 mg sodium
STAR NUTRIENTS: folate (42% DV), thiamin (21% DV), vitamin A (51% DV), vitamin B6 (14% DV), vitamin C (71% DV), vitamin K (54% DV), iron (18% DV), magnesium (13% DV), manganese (10% DV), potassium (13% DV), zinc (11% DV)

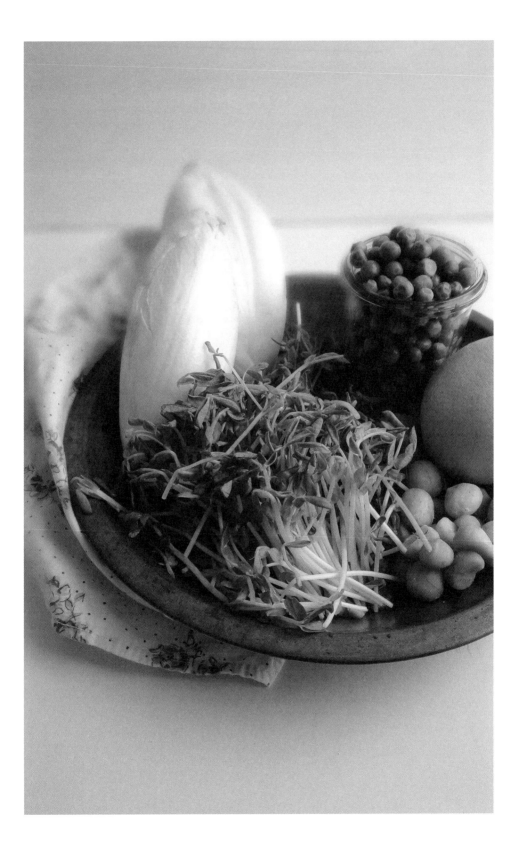

See photo
on page 88

mediterranean eggplant and artichoke lasagna

ACTIVE PREPARATION TIME: **20 minutes** • TOTAL PREPARATION TIME: **1 hour 44 minutes**

With the help of a few pantry staples—whole grain lasagna noodles, canned tomatoes and artichokes, and dried herbs—combined with fresh produce, you can whip up this vegetable lasagna with a different spin. Instead of the thick, saucy layers you'll find in classic lasagnas, this Mediterranean version focuses on roasted vegetables and a crunchy bread-crumb topping, sans the sauce. The result is a flavorful dish that boasts the warm, sunny flavors of the Mediterranean: basil, eggplant, artichokes, bell peppers, garlic. Here's a little bit of trivia: In some Mediterranean countries it was considered a crime to throw out old bread. So home cooks always saved stale bread to toast into bread crumbs, which made the simplest foods—soups, vegetables, and of course pasta—sing with texture and flavor.

MAKES 8 SERVINGS
(1 square each)

1 medium (548 g) eggplant, with peel, diced
1 medium onion, diced
1 large red bell pepper, diced
3 medium garlic cloves, minced
1½ tablespoons basil-infused extra virgin olive oil (see Notes)
1 tablespoon balsamic vinegar
1 teaspoon low-sodium herbal seasoning blend (see page 345)
¼ teaspoon freshly ground black pepper
One 14.5-ounce (411 g) can diced tomatoes, no salt added, with liquid
One 14-ounce (397 g) can artichoke hearts, in water, drained and sliced
¼ cup (10 g) chopped fresh basil, or 2 teaspoons dried
½ cup (119 ml) water
12 dry whole wheat lasagna noodles (¾ of a 9-ounce box, or 191 g total)
1 cup (112 g) shredded mozzarella-flavored plant-based cheese
¼ cup (17 g) whole grain bread crumbs (see Notes)

1. Preheat the oven to 400°F (205°C).

2. Spread the eggplant, onion, bell pepper, and garlic on a large baking sheet and drizzle with the olive oil and vinegar. Sprinkle with the herbal seasoning and black pepper. Stir well, then roast for 30 minutes. Halfway through cooking time, stir the vegetables.

3. After 30 minutes, remove the baking sheet from the oven and reduce the heat to 350°F (180°C). Add the tomatoes with their liquid, artichoke hearts, and fresh basil to the eggplant mixture on the sheet and toss to distribute.

4. Add the water to a deep 9 by 13-inch baking dish. Arrange 4 lasagna noodles along the bottom, overlapping. Spoon one-third of the vegetable mixture over the noodles, then sprinkle with ⅓ cup of the plant-based cheese. Repeat for a total of three layers.

5. Sprinkle the top layer with the prepared bread crumbs and cover with foil. Bake, covered, for 45 minutes. Remove the foil and bake for an additional 10 to 15 minutes, until the top is golden brown.

notes: You may use prepared basil-infused olive oil, available at many supermarkets and gourmet food shops, or stir ¼ teaspoon ground basil into 1½ tablespoons olive oil.

To make your own whole grain bread crumbs, toast whole grain bread (gluten-free, if desired) for 10 to 15 minutes in a 400°F (205°C) oven, until dry and brown (use 1 slice to make about ¼ cup of crumbs). Remove and let cool slightly, then place in a blender or small food processor and process into crumbs. You may do this while the vegetables are roasting (and make extra to store for another dish, if desired).

variations: You may substitute 3 small summer squashes (e.g., zucchini, crookneck, scallop) for the eggplant in step 2. To make this recipe gluten-free, use gluten-free bread crumbs, lasagna noodles, and plant-based cheese.

PER SERVING: 221 calories, 11 g protein, 32 g carbohydrate, 7 g fat, 2 g saturated fat, 8 g fiber, 6 g sugar, 286 mg sodium
STAR NUTRIENTS: niacin (11% DV), thiamin (11% DV), vitamin C (83% DV), calcium (16% DV), iron (11% DV), manganese (15% DV), potassium (10% DV)

sicilian-style eye of the goat beans

ACTIVE PREPARATION TIME: **9 minutes** • TOTAL PREPARATION TIME: **1 hour 40 minutes**
(not including soaking time)

Look to a natural food store—in the legume aisle or self-service bins—to find an array of heirloom beans—with an astonishing array of colors, shapes, sizes, flavors, and textures. You can stock up on these economical staples in your pantry, where they will last for months and inspire your wholesome, plant-powered meals. In particular, the beans in this recipe really do resemble the eye of a goat. Prepared in a simple coastal Sicilian style, with capers, olives, lemon, and oregano, this is an easy meal to throw in your slow cooker before you go to work. And when you get home you'll be greeted with a fragrant, hearty bean dish that can be paired with rustic whole grain bread and a simple green salad.

MAKES 8 SERVINGS
(about 1 cup each)

12 ounces (340 g) dried eye of the goat beans (1¾ cups; see Notes)
4 cups (948 ml) water, plus more for soaking
2 cups (474 ml) reduced sodium vegetable broth (see page 346)
One 14.5-ounce (411 g) can diced tomatoes, no salt added, with liquid
1 medium onion, diced
3 medium garlic cloves, minced
½ cup (64 g) Sicilian or Mediterranean olives, whole, drained
¼ cup (32 g) capers, drained and rinsed
Juice of ½ lemon
½ teaspoon smoked paprika
¼ teaspoon freshly ground black pepper
2 tablespoons chopped fresh oregano, or 1½ teaspoons dried

1. Cover the beans with water and soak overnight.
2. Drain the beans and add them to a large pot with the water, broth, and tomatoes. Stir well, cover, and bring to a boil over high heat.
3. Add the onion, garlic, olives, capers, lemon juice, paprika, black pepper, and oregano, cover the pot, and reduce heat to medium. Cook for about 1½ hours, until the beans are tender, stirring occasionally. Replace water lost to evaporation as needed. Serve immediately.

notes: If you cannot find eye of the goat beans, you can substitute dried large red kidney beans.

To prepare in a slow cooker, follow step 1 and drain the beans. Then add the soaked beans and all remaining ingredients to the slow cooker. Cook on high for 4 to 5 hours or on low for 8 to 10 hours, until all ingredients are tender.

If desired, you may sprinkle za'atar over the finished beans to add zing. (See page 345 to make your own.)

PER SERVING: 179 calories, 12 g protein, 31 g carbohydrate, 1.5 g fat, 0 g saturated fat, 12 g fiber, 5 g sugar, 410 mg sodium
STAR NUTRIENTS: folate (43% DV), thiamin (12% DV), vitamin C (21% DV), iron (23% DV), magnesium (16% DV), phosphorus (16% DV), potassium (17% DV)

Strawberry-Macadamia
Shortcake

For whole plant treasures, try a farmers market, CSA, or even your backyard.

Strawberry-Macadamia Shortcake
Roasted Lemon-Dill Asparagus and Tofu

Have you ever noticed that when you walk down the produce aisle of many supermarkets, you can barely detect a whiff of any scent? Yet, if you've ever picked fresh tomatoes, strawberries, or garlic, you know how intoxicating their aromas can be. The smells can hang on your hands, clothes, and hair for hours.

At your local farmers market, you can smell the ripe peaches and strawberries before you even see them displayed on tables. The reason the fruits and vegetables smell—and taste—so wonderful is that they are often picked perfectly ripe just hours before the farmers take them to the market, and they are at their flavor and nutrition peak. You'll find moist soil still clinging to the roots of potatoes and radishes, and the fresh tops of beets and carrots still intact. Buying this produce is a wonderful way to connect with local farmers, learn more about how your food is produced, and find produce grown without synthetic pesticides and fertilizers. Buying this "clean" produce supports a sustainable food system (see page 267).

This same benefit can be found in a CSA (community supported agriculture), which offers you a "share" of a local farm's bounty for a reasonable price. If you join a CSA, you'll pick up or be delivered a box of fresh, local seasonal produce once a week. The surprise variety of fruits and vegetables will encourage you to get creative and try less common plants, such as kohlrabi and rutabagas.

Don't give up on your supermarket; more of them are getting fresh and local by working with nearby farmers to supply farm-fresh, ripe produce, and some are even organizing CSAs in their parking lots. And don't forget— the freshest produce you will ever experience can be grown at home. If you have a yard, sacrifice a flower bed for vegetables, plant an apple tree, or just place a tomato plant or herb pot on your doorstep or windowsill. Revel in produce picked ripe and fresh—wherever you can find it.

See photo
on page 98

strawberry-macadamia shortcake

ACTIVE PREPARATION TIME: **16 minutes** • TOTAL PREPARATION TIME: **34 minutes**

One of my favorite ways to do desserts is to maximize the natural sweetening power of fruits. When strawberries are in season in late spring through early summer, make the most of these sweet, scarlet beauties. You'll find them fresh in supermarkets, farmers markets, and your CSA—and you can even grow them in your garden. In addition to slicing them into cereals, salads, and parfaits, turn to this classic dessert—strawberry shortcake— with my own plant-powered twist. The tender shortcakes are divine piled high with fresh strawberries, coconut topping, and a dusting of macadamia nuts.

MAKES 6 SERVINGS
(one shortcake each)

. . . .

Shortcake
Nonstick cooking spray
¾ cup (84 g) almond flour or almond meal
1½ cups (180 g) whole wheat pastry flour
1 teaspoon cinnamon
1 tablespoon baking powder
⅓ cup (84 g) soft dairy-free margarine (see Notes on page 223)
2 tablespoons agave nectar
3 tablespoons unsweetened coconut milk beverage

Topping
1 pound (454 g) fresh strawberries, sliced (3½ to 4 cups)
1 cup (227 g) vanilla- or strawberry-flavored cultured coconut
 yogurt
2 tablespoons chopped macadamia nuts

1. Preheat the oven to 375°F (190°C). Spray a baking sheet with nonstick cooking spray. In a small bowl, mix together the almond meal, whole wheat pastry flour, cinnamon, and baking powder. Cut in the margarine with a fork, then use a wooden spoon to mix in the agave and coconut milk to make a dough. Place the dough on a lightly floured surface and roll out to about 1-inch thickness. Using a 3-inch round cutter, cut out 6 shortcakes. Place the shortcakes on the baking sheet and bake for 18 to 20 minutes, until golden brown.

2. Meanwhile, to prepare the topping, place ½ cup of the sliced strawberries in a small bowl and mash them with a fork to achieve a lumpy, juicy texture. Stir the coconut yogurt into the mashed strawberries. Place remaining strawberries in a 1-quart bowl.

3. While the shortcakes are warm, slice them in half horizontally. Place each bottom half onto individual dessert plates. Top each with one sixth of the fresh strawberries (about ½ cup), one sixth of the yogurt mixture (about 2½ tablespoons), 1 teaspoon of chopped macadamia nuts, and the top half of the shortcake. Serve immediately.

variation: Substitute frozen sliced strawberries when fresh are not available. You can also substitute sliced peaches, nectarines, bananas, or mangoes for strawberries in this recipe. To make this gluten-free, substitute 1¼ cups all-purpose gluten-free flour blend (such as Bob's Red Mill or King Arthur Flour) for the 1½ cups whole wheat pastry flour and check that all other ingredients are gluten-free.

PER SERVING: 291 calories, 6 g protein, 32 g carbohydrate, 16 g fat, 3 g saturated fat, 7 g fiber, 7 g sugar, 15 mg sodium

STAR NUTRIENTS: thiamin (14% DV), vitamin C (72% DV), vitamin E (18% DV), calcium (13% DV), iron (15% DV), magnesium (18% DV), manganese (21% DV), zinc (11% DV)

---

roasted lemon-dill asparagus and tofu

ACTIVE PREPARATION TIME: **7 minutes** • TOTAL PREPARATION TIME: **37 minutes**

Asparagus is one of spring's most celebrated plants—as the young spears push up to greet the warming sun, they bring forth a delicate flavor. Yet this subtle vegetable is packed with nutrition—fiber, vitamins, minerals, and antioxidants linked with heart and anti-cancer benefits. Look for fresh asparagus in your local supermarket and farmers market. It's a great addition to your garden—plant it once and it will come up in the same spot for the next 20 years. Roasting the whole asparagus is one of my favorite preparation styles—especially served with lemon zest and fresh dill as this recipe calls for.

MAKES 4 SERVINGS
(about 6 asparagus spears and 2 ounces of tofu each)

One 12-ounce (340 g) bunch fresh asparagus (about 24 spears), ends trimmed
8 ounces (227 g) extra firm tofu, drained, pressed for best results (see Note), and cubed
Juice and zest of 1 small lemon
2 teaspoons extra virgin olive oil
1 teaspoon Dijon mustard
1 medium garlic clove, minced
¼ teaspoon white pepper
Pinch of sea salt, optional
¼ cup (15 g) chopped fresh dill, or ½ teaspoon dried

1. Preheat the oven to 375°F (190°C).
2. Arrange the asparagus on the bottom of a 9 by 13-inch baking dish and top with the tofu.
3. In a small dish, whisk together the lemon juice, olive oil, mustard, garlic, white pepper, and sea salt, if desired, and pour onto the asparagus.
4. Place the dish in the oven on the top rack and roast for 30 to 35 minutes, until the asparagus is crisp-tender and slightly browned. Stir halfway through cooking.
5. Remove the dish from the oven, sprinkle with the dill and lemon zest, and serve immediately.

note: For best results, you may want to press the tofu, which decreases the moisture and promotes a springy texture that absorbs more flavor in dishes. To press a block of firm or extra firm tofu, wrap it in four layers of paper towels and place on a plate. Cover with another plate and top with a heavy item, such as a large book, so that the tofu is pressed down. Set aside for 30 minutes to drain. Remove the tofu and discard paper towels. You may repeat a second time for an even drier consistency. You can also freeze tofu as another way to remove moisture, but this will change the texture slightly (thaw before using in a dish).

Another option is to invest in a tofu press, which speeds up the process. This handy tool is becoming more and more popular, and inexpensive brands are available at specialty kitchen supplies stores and online.

variation: You may omit the tofu for a lighter side dish.

PER SERVING: 97 calories, 8 g protein, 8 g carbohydrate, 6 g fat, .5 g saturated fat, 3 g fiber, 3 g sugar, 37 mg sodium
STAR NUTRIENTS: folate (14% DV), vitamin A (14% DV), vitamin C (44% DV), vitamin K (13% DV), calcium (14% DV), iron (17% DV), magnesium (11% DV)

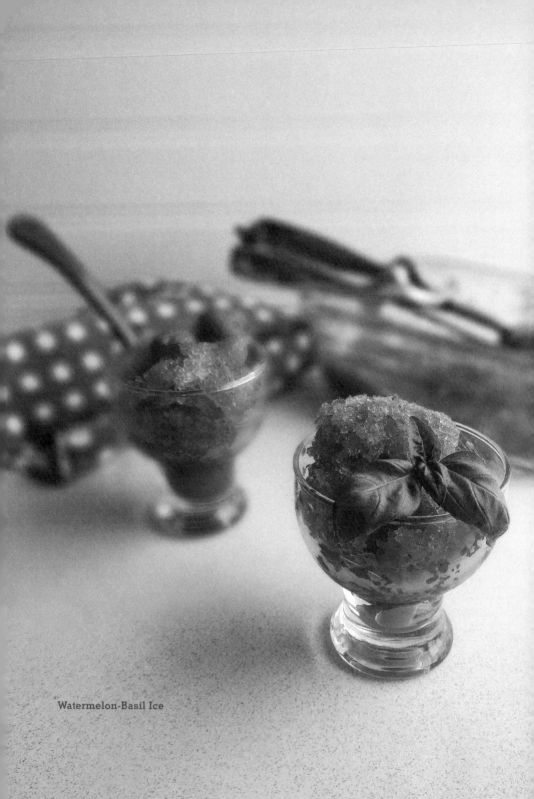

Watermelon-Basil Ice

Shoot for three to four servings of fruit a day.

Watermelon-Basil Ice
Peach and Cranberry Crumble

Mother Nature must be really proud of one of her finest accomplishments: fruits. These naturally sweet plants come in all shapes, sizes, and colors, with an array of textures, flavors, and aromas. Just close your eyes and imagine strawberries, and saliva will flow to your tongue as you recall the unique, sweet, floral taste and aroma that is the calling card of this fruit. The same will occur with other fruits we have grown to love.

Even though we have such an amazing variety of fruits that are available to us, from tropical pineapple to forest berries, we fall short on eating enough of them. It's a pity, because they are densely packed with disease-protective nutrients, such as fiber, vitamin C, vitamin A, potassium, and more. They also owe the bright colors of their skins, flesh, and seeds to phytochemicals, which, as you've learned, hold tremendous significance for protecting our health. For example, peaches—rich in beta-carotene—appear to protect the heart, and citrus fruits—plump with liminoids—may help fight cancer.

Nearly every culture throughout history has celebrated local fruits and enjoyed these precious plants all year by preserving them, from dried mangoes in India to applesauce in Eastern Europe (see page 343). In order to gain the maximal health benefits related to eating fruit, meet your goal of three to four servings per day—whether from fresh, canned, frozen, or dried (without added sugar). Choose whole pieces of fruit, not fruit juice, which has been condensed into a beverage low in fiber, high in glycemic index (see page 000), and dense in natural sugars that can produce rapid rises of glucose in your bloodstream. Include a serving of fruit at each meal and as a snack to power up on these vital—and delicious—plants.

See photo
on page 104

watermelon-basil ice

ACTIVE PREPARATION TIME: 6 minutes • TOTAL PREPARATION TIME: 3 to 4 hours

It's easy to fit in more fruits when they look, smell, and taste like this!
All this dessert consists of is ripe watermelon, fresh basil, and a twist of
lemon, yet this wholesome fruit sorbet offers a cool treat on a summer day,
or a nice palate cleanser after a hearty meal.

MAKES 6 SERVINGS
(about ⅔ cup each)

6 cups (654) cubed fresh ripe watermelon
½ cup (20 g) packed fresh basil leaves
1 tablespoon lemon juice

1. Place the watermelon, basil, and lemon juice in a blender. Process just until smooth.
2. Pour the mixture into a shallow airtight freezer container. For best results, freeze for 3 to 4 hours until the texture is frozen yet scoopable. Use a metal ice cream scoop to portion into serving dishes.
3. Freeze any leftovers. To serve again, thaw at room temperature for about 10 minutes before scooping.

variation: Substitute cantaloupe, peaches, or strawberries for the watermelon.

PER SERVING: 46 calories, 1 g protein, 12 g carbohydrate, 0 g fat, 0 g saturated fat,
1 g fiber, 9 g sugar, 2 mg sodium
STAR NUTRIENTS: vitamin A (20% DV), vitamin C (23% DV)

peach and cranberry crumble

ACTIVE PREPARATION TIME: **12 minutes** • TOTAL PREPARATION TIME: **52 minutes**

This is my go-to fruit-based dessert. It takes just minutes to whip up this peach-cranberry crumble, yet your kitchen will smell wonderful as the baked cinnamon aroma fills it with sweet warmth. Plus, you'll gain another serving of disease-fighting fruit in your day. During the winter, turn to canned peaches as a foolproof substitute for fresh.

MAKES 6 SERVINGS
(2 peach halves each)

6 ripe fresh peaches, halved, or two 15.25-ounce (432 g) jars
   no-sugar-added peach halves in juice, drained, juice reserved (see Notes)
½ cup (53 g) dried cranberries
½ cup juice (reserved from canned peaches, or 100% peach or
   apple juice)
½ cup (60 g) white whole wheat flour
¾ cup (117 g) uncooked old-fashioned oats
½ teaspoon cinnamon
¼ teaspoon allspice
¼ teaspoon nutmeg
1½ tablespoons light brown sugar or coconut palm sugar
¼ cup (29 g) chopped walnuts
3 tablespoons soft dairy-free margarine (see Notes on page 000)

1. Preheat the oven to 375°F (190°C).
2. Place the peaches (hollow side facing down) on the bottom of a 9 by 13-inch baking dish.
3. Sprinkle with the dried cranberries.
4. Pour the juice over the fruit.
5. In a medium bowl, stir the flour, oats, cinnamon, allspice, nutmeg, brown sugar, and walnuts together. Cut in the margarine to form a crumbly mixture.
6. Sprinkle the oat mixture evenly over the top of the fruit.
7. Place the dish in the oven and bake for about 40 minutes, until the fruit is tender and the top is golden.
8. Serve warm.

recipe continues

notes: If you use canned peaches, cut down the baking time by 10 minutes. This is excellent served with plant-based vanilla ice cream.

variations: Substitute fresh apples or pears for the peaches. To make this gluten-free, substitute an all-purpose gluten-free flour blend (such as Bob's Red Mill or King Arthur Flour) for the whole wheat flour and check that all other ingredients, especially the oats, are gluten-free.

PER SERVING: 266 calories, 4 g protein, 42 g carbohydrate, 10 g fat, 2 g saturated fat, 5 g fiber, 24 g sugar, 68 mg sodium

STAR NUTRIENTS: niacin (10% DV), vitamin A (14% DV), vitamin C (16% DV), vitamin E (10% DV), manganese (36% DV), potassium (10% DV), selenium (10% DV)

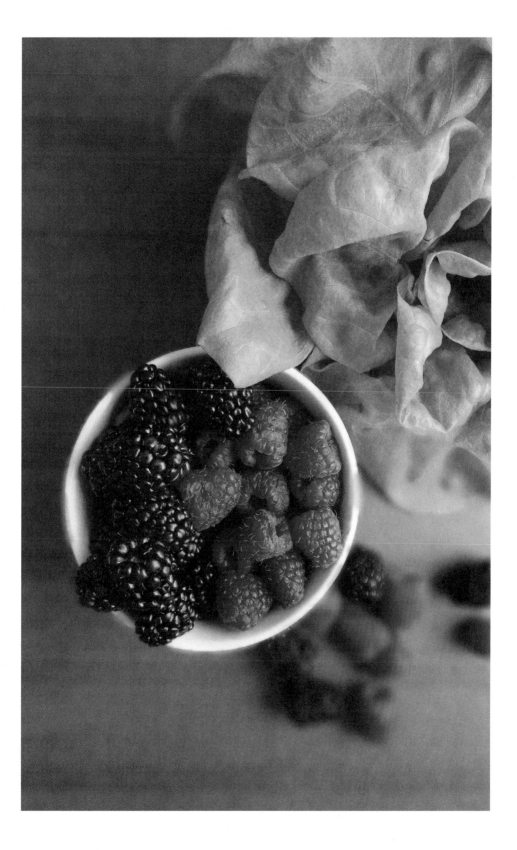

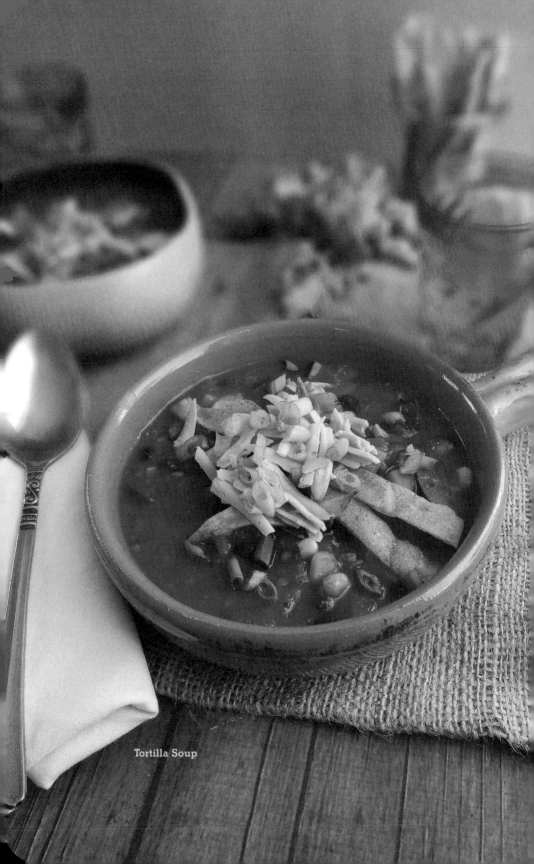

Tortilla Soup

Remember, fresh isn't always best.

Tortilla Soup
Fig Oat Bars

Usually when you read about the health benefits of fruits and vegetables in a magazine or on the Internet, you also find the word *fresh*. In fact, surveys show that people favor fresh produce so much that many don't even count canned fruits and vegetables as servings! But this kind of thinking is just wrong. We've been preserving precious plant foods since the dawn of time—drying fruits, vegetables, and grains in the sun; fermenting vegetables into pickles; and, later on, canning or freezing produce at its peak.

Please, enjoy fresh produce when it's available. Eat your fill of berries, stone fruit, corn, and green beans during the summer season. But as the season fades away, turn to canned, frozen, and dried produce more often, which are much more sustainable options than fresh produce not in season. They still contribute servings of fruits and vegetables to your day, as well as important nutrients. Although some nutrients, such as fiber and vitamins C and B, may be a bit lower in preserved produce, other nutrients may be even higher. For example, the antioxidant lycopene is even higher in canned tomatoes. During canning, fruits and vegetables are heated, which may increase the availability of certain nutrients in some plants, like tomatoes, because the cell walls in the plant are disrupted, releasing the nutrients to be absorbed more readily.

It's easy to see why you should rely on preserved produce in your plant-powered diet when you consider their nutrition, ripe flavor, ease of use, and economical price. Stock your pantry with canned unsalted beans, tomatoes, peaches, pineapple, and corn to add to soups, salads, side dishes, fruit desserts, and main dishes. Gather a selection of dried, unsweetened fruits such as berries, pears, raisins, figs, and dates for snacks, baking, and cereal toppings. Try dried tomatoes and mushrooms as flavor enhancers. Fill your freezer with frozen, unsweetened fruits for smoothies and cereal and yogurt toppings, as well as vegetables like edamame, green beans, spinach, and peas for salads, soups, and side dishes. Best of all, these preserved fruits and vegetables are a cinch to use—no washing or chopping required.

See photo
on page 110

tortilla soup

ACTIVE PREPARATION TIME: **24 minutes** • TOTAL PREPARATION TIME: **48 minutes**

A traditional Mexican dish, tortilla soup is a spicy blend of tomatoes, vegetables, and crisp tortilla strips. This easy plant-powered version—you can whip it up in no time—throws protein-rich black beans into the mix. Best of all, this dish relies on preserved goods, such as canned tomatoes, frozen corn, and canned beans, so you can make it year-round from your pantry. And it's a great complement for a simple sandwich, burrito, or vegetable salad for lunch or dinner.

MAKES 10 SERVINGS
(generous 1 cup each)

Tortilla Strips
Three 6-inch (15 cm) corn tortillas
2 teaspoons extra virgin olive oil
½ teaspoon chili powder

Soup
4 teaspoons extra virgin olive oil
1 medium onion, diced
1 medium garlic clove, minced
1 medium green bell pepper, diced
1 small jalapeño pepper, finely diced
1 small zucchini, diced
1 cup (164 g) frozen corn
¼ teaspoon crushed red pepper
2 teaspoons cumin
4 cups (948 ml) water
1 tablespoon reduced sodium vegetable broth base
Two 14.5-ounce (411 g) cans diced tomatoes, with liquid
One 15-ounce (425 g) can black beans, with liquid (or 1¾ cups
   cooked, with ½ cup water)
⅔ cup (37 g) plant-based cheese, optional
⅔ cup (60 g) chopped green onions, white and green parts

1. Preheat the oven to 400°F (205°C).
2. Slice the tortillas into thin strips. Place them on a baking sheet and drizzle with 2 teaspoons of olive oil, then sprinkle the chili powder on top. Bake for about 5 to 8 minutes, until brown and crisp. Remove from oven and set aside. Turn off the oven.
3. Meanwhile, prepare the soup by heating the remaining 2 teaspoons of olive oil in a large pot over medium heat. Add the onion and sauté for 5 minutes.

4. Add the garlic, bell pepper, jalapeño, zucchini, corn, crushed red pepper, and cumin and sauté for an additional 5 minutes.

5. Add the water, broth base, tomatoes, and black beans. Stir well and cover. Simmer over medium heat for 25 to 30 minutes, until vegetables are tender.

6. Ladle about 1 cup of soup into soup bowls, and garnish with a few tortilla strips, 1 tablespoon of plant-based cheese, and 1 tablespoon green onions. Serve immediately.

7. Store leftover soup (without garnishes) in the refrigerator for up to 3 days. Reheat the soup and garnish with the tortilla strips, cheese, and green onions.

variation: Substitute cooked or canned white beans, pinto beans, garbanzo beans, or kidney beans for black beans, or use a combination.

PER SERVING: 148 calories, 5 g protein, 21 g carbohydrate, 5 g fat, 1 g saturated fat, 5 g fiber, 5 g sugar, 263 mg sodium
STAR NUTRIENTS: folate (12% DV), vitamin A (13%), vitamin C (40% DV), calcium (14% DV), manganese (11% DV), molybdenum (44% DV), phosphorus (10% DV), potassium (10% DV)

fig oat bars

A perfect treat for kids' (and grown-ups'!) lunch boxes, this rich, gooey fig bar is packed with whole grain, nut, and fruit goodness. And since it relies on preserved foods, such as dried fruits, you can keep these ingredients on hand to whip up this dessert in minutes. It's great served warm with a steaming cup of coffee on a chilly day. Plus, it's packed with health-protective fiber and phytochemicals, such as anthocyanin—the bioactive plant compound responsible for the purple-black color in figs and linked to benefits, such as brain health.

MAKES 16 SERVINGS
(one 2 by 2-inch square each)

4 ounces (120 g) dried figs, such as Black Mission
⅔ cup (156 ml) water
Nonstick cooking spray
1 cup (120 g) white whole wheat flour
½ cup (56 g) almond flour or almond meal
½ cup (78 g) uncooked old-fashioned oats
¼ cup (54 g) chopped almonds
½ teaspoon baking soda
1 teaspoon cinnamon
¼ cup (59 ml) canola oil, expeller pressed
¼ cup (59 ml) unsweetened plain plant-based milk
2 tablespoon maple syrup
Zest of 1 small lemon

1. Place the figs in a small pot with water and cover. Bring to a boil over medium heat and cook for 1 minute, then turn off the heat and leave the figs in the pot, covered, to rest for 10 minutes.
2. Preheat the oven to 350°F (180°C). Spray an 8 by 8-inch baking dish with nonstick cooking spray.
3. Meanwhile, mix the white whole wheat flour, almond flour, oats, almonds, baking soda, and cinnamon together. Stir in the canola oil, plant-based milk, and maple syrup to make a dough.
4. Place the figs with their liquid and the lemon zest into a blender and process into a thick paste. Pause to scrape down the sides of the blender as needed.
5. Pat about two thirds of the dough into the bottom of the dish. Spread the fig paste on top. Scatter the remaining dough over it in small crumbs. Bake for 25 to 30 minutes, until golden brown.

6. Allow to cool for 10 minutes, then slice into 16 squares. Serve immediately.

note: Store leftover bars in an airtight container in the refrigerator for up to one week.

variation: Substitute raisins, prunes, or dried apricots for figs, or use a combination. To make this gluten-free, substitute an all-purpose gluten-free flour blend (such as Bob's Red Mill or King Authur Flour) for the white whole wheat flour and check that all other ingredients are gluten-free.

PER SERVING: 135 calories, 3 g protein, 20 g carbohydrate, 6 g fat, .5 g saturated fat, 10 g sugar, 6 mg sodium
STAR NUTRIENTS: riboflavin (11% DV)

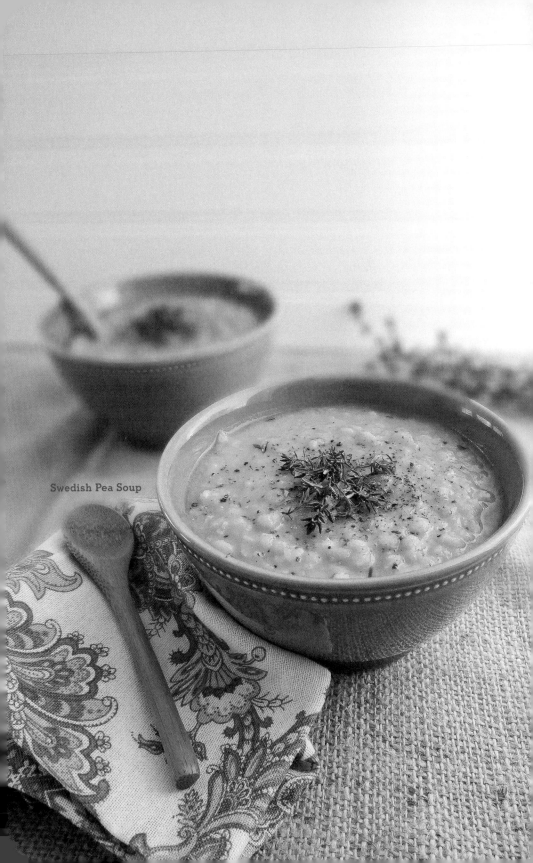

Swedish Pea Soup

Be globally inspired.

Swedish Pea Soup
Pesto Trapanese with Whole Grain Penne

We're so lucky to live in the modern world, where the sheer volume of foods available is staggering—the United States alone produces about 350 billion pounds of food each year (about twice as much as needed!). With the exchange of plants over the past several centuries, people around the world can benefit from the diverse cultivation of plant foods, from the sun-craving (like grapes, olives, and citrus) to the cold-loving (such as wheat and apples), and everything in between.

Add to that the enormous ethnic diversity in major cities across the globe, which gives rise to a wide variety of cuisines from all over the world. In many cities, you can enjoy authentic Thai, Middle Eastern, Mexican, Italian, French, Indian, and Chinese any day of the week. Modern "comfort foods" include tacos, spaghetti, or Chinese stir-fry. Flavors from different food cultures are even woven together to redefine traditional foods—the fusion trend that is still going strong. And now the food world is getting even smaller, as people incorporate even farther-afield locations into their culinary food lexicon, from Ethiopian to Vietnamese to Malaysian.

Today's affinity for global flavors creates an exciting path to more flavorful plant foods. Most ethnic cuisines from around the world have a firm footing in plant-based cooking, from Caribbean beans and rice to Korean spicy vegetable soups with tofu. We can learn so much about cooking delicious, flavorful plant-powered dishes by infusing our foods with global flavor. Borrow a trick from Puerto Rican kitchens and start off your bean dishes with *sofrito*—a zesty cooking base made with cilantro, annatto, green peppers, and garlic (see page 200). Infuse your whole grains with abundant flavor by trying the Lebanese culinary tradition of tabbouleh, tossing grains with mint, parsley, tomatoes, and garlic (see page 164). I have borrowed upon the world's melting pot of flavors to inspire my plant-powered recipes. Bon appétit (or *buon appetito*, or *buen provecho*)!

See photo
on page 116

swedish pea soup

ACTIVE PREPARATION TIME: **7 minutes** • TOTAL PREPARATION TIME: **1 hour 30 minutes to 2 hours** (not including soaking)

Every country has its own plant-based food traditions, including the northerly country of Sweden, where my husband hails from. Pea soup dates back to ancient Roman times, when it was a nutritious, peasant food staple, but it eventually became one of the time-honored foods of Sweden. Ärtsoppa (pea soup) has been traditionally served in homes, schools, and restaurants every Thursday, along with thin, crepelike pancakes, for hundreds of years. Made with yellow peas, this simple soup is prepared with sweet, zesty mustard. Pea soup's hallowed history is justified by the nutrition brimming in each bowl: 14 grams of protein, and a good source of several essential nutrients.

MAKES 8 SERVINGS
(almost 1 cup each)

1 pound (454 g) dried yellow peas (see Notes)
6 cups (1,420 ml) water
1 medium onion, diced
1 tablespoon reduced sodium vegetable broth base
1 tablespoon prepared mustard (e.g., Swedish, whole grain, or
    Dijon; see Notes)
½ teaspoon freshly ground black pepper
1 teaspoon low-sodium herbal seasoning blend (see page 345)
1 bay leaf
1 teaspoon marjoram
1 teaspoon thyme

1. Cover the dried yellow peas with water and soak overnight.
2. Drain the peas and place them in a large heavy pot.
3. Add the remaining ingredients, stir well, cover with a lid, and bring to a boil over high heat. Reduce the heat to medium and simmer for 1½ to 2 hours, stirring occasionally, until the peas are tender. Add water as needed to replace moisture lost to evaporation. Remove the bay leaf before serving.

notes: Traditional Swedish pea soup uses whole yellow peas (not split). If you are unable to find whole yellow peas, substitute split yellow peas, but reduce the cooking time by about 30 minutes, as they will cook faster.

Swedish mustard (*senap*), which may be found in some gourmet and international shops, has a characteristic sweet yet spicy flavor.

To make this in a slow cooker, soak and drain the peas, then combine with the other ingredients and cook for 4 to 6 hours on high or 8 to 10 hours on low.

PER SERVING: 203 calories, 14 g protein, 36 g carbohydrate, 1 g fat, 0 g saturated fat, 15 g fiber, 5 g sugar, 59 mg sodium

STAR NUTRIENTS: folate (39% DV), thiamin (28% DV), calcium (10% DV), iron (16% DV), magnesium (17% DV), potassium (16% DV), zinc (12% DV)

pesto trapanese with whole grain penne

ACTIVE PREPARATION TIME: **11 minutes** • TOTAL PREPARATION TIME: **18 minutes**

You can learn many lessons about plant-powered food in the Mediterranean. On my trip to the Sicilian island Pantelleria, I was lucky enough to learn how to prepare this traditional dish at the side of a local chef. He explained that pesto trapanese is classic Sicilian peasant food, which is all about "creating something from nothing." Those "nothing" ingredients include almonds, garlic, basil, tomatoes, olive oil, and pasta. It's amazing how simple and delicious this dish is—it's the perfect solution for a 30-minute meal made of ingredients you can keep on hand. My Pantellerian chef hammered the rough pesto with the help of an enormous terra-cotta mortar and pestle, which you can find in gourmet kitchen shops. If you don't want to invest in one, you can use modern equipment, such as a food processor, which makes the job a lot easier.

MAKES 6 SERVINGS
(about ¾ cup each)

⅓ cup (31 g) finely chopped almonds
8 ounces (227 g) uncooked whole grain penne
4 medium garlic cloves
1½ tablespoons extra virgin olive oil
2 cups (48 g) packed fresh basil leaves
2 cups (about 10 ounces, 284 g) quartered fresh cherry tomatoes, room temperature (see Notes)
¼ teaspoon freshly ground black pepper
Pinch of sea salt, optional

1. Preheat the oven to 350°F (180°F).
2. Place the almonds in a small ovenproof dish and toast for about 5 minutes, just until brown (see Notes). Remove from the oven and set aside.
3. Meanwhile, fill a medium pot with water, cover, and bring to a boil over high heat. Add the pasta, reduce the heat to medium, and cook for about 8 minutes, until al dente. Drain, return to the pot, and cover to keep warm.
4. While the pasta is cooking, combine the garlic and olive oil in a food processor or blender. Process for just a few seconds, until creamy.
5. Add the basil leaves, tomatoes, and black pepper. Process just until pesto is chopped (5 to 10 seconds). Do not overprocess; the mixture should be chunky, not completely pureed. Taste and add sea salt, if desired.

6. Add the pesto to the hot pasta and toss. Transfer to a serving platter and sprinkle with the toasted almonds and serve immediately.

notes: You may also toast the almonds—stirring constantly—in a skillet over medium-high heat for 3 to 5 minutes.

This pesto is fresh and is not heated. Thus, it's important to use room-temperature, not refrigerated ingredients, and to have the pesto ready to go as soon as the pasta is cooked so that the dish doesn't get cold.

PER SERVING: 222 calories, 10 g protein, 34 g carbohydrate, 7 g fat, 1 g saturated fat, 6 g fiber, 2 g sugar, 9 mg sodium
STAR NUTRIENTS: folate (21% DV), niacin (16% DV), riboflavin (11% DV), thiamin (10% DV), vitamin A (88% DV), vitamin C (35% DV), vitamin E (13% DV), vitamin K (398% DV), calcium (17% DV), copper (28% DV), iron (23% DV), magnesium (31% DV), manganese (112% DV), phosphorus (18% DV), potassium (13% DV), zinc (12% DV)

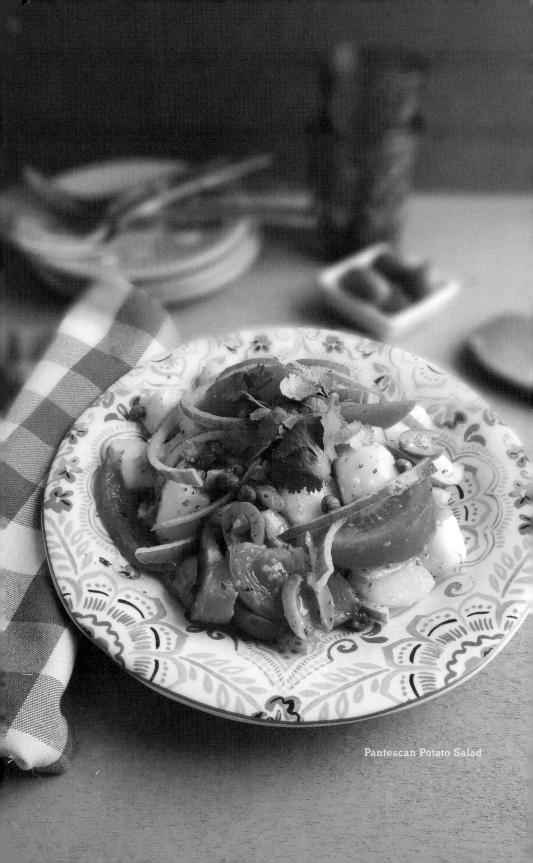

Pantescan Potato Salad

Make the switch to extra virgin olive oil.

Pantescan Potato Salad
Roasted Cauliflower with Freshly Ground Spices

Simply pressed olive oil, obtained in ancient times by crushing olives against stones to collect the precious oil, has been considered a health tonic throughout the ages. And now science confirms that extra virgin olive oil, one of the least refined plant oils, is rich in heart-healthy monounsaturated fats, and anti-inflammatory and antioxidant compounds. Perhaps because of this, extra virgin olive oil (a key feature in the much-praised Mediterranean diet) has been linked by a body of research with protection against heart disease, and studies are also pointing out potential protection against breast cancer.

Extra virgin olive oil is not only good for you, but it makes everything *taste* good, too. Just a drizzle over your salad, veggies, whole grains, and legumes can ramp up their flavor, and their nutrition, too—the fat helps your body absorb the antioxidants in vegetables. Make this the number one oil in your kitchen for dressings and marinades, cooking, and even baking.

Just remember that olive oil—like all fats—is a concentrated source of energy. At 120 calories per tablespoon, it's easy to pour on the calories when you glug on the olive oil. If you're watching your weight, a teaspoon (about 40 calories) of olive oil is plenty for taste and health. Try using a mister (or spray bottle) or a spout to control the volume. My favorite way to cook vegetables is à la Mediterranean: sauté any vegetables with a touch of olive oil, a small amount of water, crushed garlic, and some herbs and spices, such as oregano, basil, or paprika, until they are crisp-tender. You can also borrow another Mediterranean trick for salads: scrap the bottled dressings and just drizzle tiny amounts of olive oil and vinegar directly onto your salad. The taste is clean and simple, and your table will look great with a cruet set (available at kitchen and home goods stores) as a centerpiece.

Extra virgin olive oil is also one of the most minimally processed vegetable oils on the market; standards require that the oil is obtained from olives without any treatments that impact the oil in any way, such as using solvents or washing the oil. That's why its bioactive compounds remain intact. However, you may not want the strong taste of olives flavoring some foods, such as baked goods. So, in these cases, I suggest canola oil because of its similar heart-healthy fat profile. The best types of vegetable oils are expeller pressed, which means that no petroleum products are used to extract the oils.

pantescan potato salad

See photo
on page 122

ACTIVE PREPARATION TIME: **12 minutes** • TOTAL PREPARATION TIME: **35 minutes**

On my trip to Pantelleria, I fell in love with the rustic, authentic Mediterranean food, which featured plant foods grown locally on the island. This simple potato salad, infused with flavors of olives and capers, was served at almost every meal. The heart-healthy fats found in extra virgin olive oil are a key feature of the Mediterranean diet and provide a mountain of health benefits.

MAKES 8 SERVINGS
(1 cup each)

3 medium potatoes, peeled if desired
4 cups (948 ml) water
4 large tomatoes, sliced into wedges
½ medium red or sweet onion, halved and sliced into rings
½ cup (64 g) Sicilian olives, drained (see Note)
1½ tablespoons capers, drained and rinsed
1½ tablespoons extra virgin olive oil
1½ teaspoons red wine vinegar
1½ teaspoons dried oregano

1. Place the potatoes and water in a pot, cover, and bring to a boil over medium-high heat. Reduce the heat to medium and cook until tender but firm, about 25 minutes. Drain, remove, and let cool.

2. Slice the potatoes into large chunks and place them in a large bowl with the tomatoes, onions, olives, and capers. Toss together.

3. Drizzle with the olive oil and vinegar and add the oregano. Toss to combine well. Serve immediately. (This salad is good served at room temperature or chilled.)

note: Sicilian olives may be available at specialty food stores, often at an olive bar. If unavailable, substitute kalamata olives.

PER SERVING: 148 calories, 3 g protein, 26 g carbohydrate, 4.5 g fat, .5 g saturated fat, 4 g fiber, 4 g sugar, 162 mg sodium
STAR NUTRIENTS: niacin (10% DV), vitamin A (17% DV), vitamin B6 (18% DV), vitamin C (35% DV), manganese (12% DV), potassium (16% DV)

roasted cauliflower with freshly ground spices

ACTIVE PREPARATION TIME: **8 minutes** • TOTAL PREPARATION TIME: **48 minutes**

Roasting vegetables is a delicious and healthful way to ramp up flavor, as well as nutrition. Studies show that when vegetables are prepared deliciously, with a touch of olive oil, people end up eating more vegetables. And cauliflower is part of the brassica family, chock-full of intriguing sulfur compounds linked with cancer protection. Paired with freshly ground Indian spices, this simple side dish shimmers with warm, golden aromas and flavors. Serve it with Bell Pepper Rye Pilaf (page 54) and some simple simmered lentils and you've got a comfort meal that will satisfy a whole army, for such a small cost.

MAKES 8 SERVINGS
(about ⅔ cup each)

1 medium head cauliflower, trimmed and broken into medium-size florets (about 5 cups or 575 g; see Note)
1½ tablespoons extra virgin olive oil
1 tablespoon lemon juice
3 cardamom pods
¼ teaspoon crushed red pepper
¼ teaspoon black peppercorns
½ teaspoon coriander seeds
½ teaspoon cumin seeds

1. Preheat the oven to 400°F (205°C).
2. Spread the cauliflower florets in a 9 by 13-inch baking dish.
3. Combine the olive oil and lemon juice in a small dish.
4. Add the cardamom pods, crushed red pepper, black peppercorns, coriander seeds, and cumin seeds to a small food processor or spice grinder. Grind into a fine powder. Add the ground spices to the olive oil mixture and toss together.
5. Pour the spice mixture over the cauliflower and toss together using clean hands to evenly distribute.
6. Place the dish in the oven, uncovered, and roast for about 40 minutes, stirring every 15 minutes, until the cauliflower is golden brown and tender.

note: Try different varieties of cauliflower, such as orange, green, or purple.

variations: Add 8 ounces (227 g) cubed extra firm tofu (pressed, for best results—see page 103) in step 2.

PER SERVING: 51 calories, 2 g protein, 6 g carbohydrate, 3 g fat, 0 g saturated fat, 2 g fiber, 1 g sugar, 32 mg sodium
STAR NUTRIENTS: folate (15% DV), pantothenic acid (19% DV), vitamin B6 (10% DV), vitamin C (86% DV), vitamin K (14% DV), manganese (13% DV)

Pumpkin Spice Muffins
with Pumpkin Seeds

Be very picky about carbs.

Pumpkin Spice Muffins with Pumpkin Seeds
Stir-Fried Barley with Sea Vegetables and Peanuts

A few decades ago, nutrition experts advised you to bulk up on carbs, with little attention to the type. Then the diet pendulum swung the other direction, as carbs became enemy number one. Today we know that it's not so much the *amount* of carbs that causes problems as the *type*. Turns out that feasting on quickly digestible, refined carbs—such as snack foods, sugary treats and beverages, and white bread made with refined flour—is not such a healthy thing. These high-glycemic foods, stripped of many nutrients and fiber, are readily absorbed and digested in the body, sharply raising your blood glucose levels. A diet filled with such carbohydrate sources has been associated with health risks, such heart disease, type 2 diabetes, and obesity.

However, when you focus instead on unrefined carbohydrates sources, such as whole plant foods in their natural form—whole grains, beans, lentils, nuts, seeds, vegetables, fruits—your body reacts differently. These low-glycemic foods—rich in fiber—take longer to digest and absorb into your bloodstream; thus, they produce slower, smaller rises in blood glucose levels, which puts less demand on your body to produce insulin (the hormone that ushers glucose from your bloodstream into your body's tissues, where it can be used for energy). They also offer the payback of a rich nutrient supply, including powerful antioxidants that help fight oxidative stress in the body, which can damage your cells and tissues.

One of *the* most important things you can do for your health is be choosier when it comes to selecting carbs. Choose whole wheat bread over white bread, brown rice over white rice, whole grain pasta over refined pasta, and wheat berries or kasha instead of packaged white rice side dish mixes. Trade highly refined breakfast cereals for whole grain porridge. Skip the processed snack crackers and chips and choose whole grain flat bread. Swap those sugary nutrition bars for homemade trail mix (see page 284). Limit your sweet treats to small servings occasionally (see page 221) and make fruit your go-to sweet fix.

See photo
on page 128

pumpkin spice muffins with pumpkin seeds

ACTIVE PREPARATION TIME: 11 minutes • TOTAL PREPARATION TIME: 55 minutes

You don't have to feel guilty about eating carbs when you choose whole grains. The addition of seeds, dates, spices, and beta-carotene-rich pumpkin packs these muffins with nutrients, antioxidants, and slow-digesting carbs. Make a batch and store them in the freezer to microwave for breakfast, snacks, or lunch or dinner alongside a soup or salad.

MAKES 12 SERVINGS
(1 muffin each)

Nonstick cooking spray
½ cup (123 g) canned or cooked pumpkin
1¼ cups (119 ml) unsweetened plain plant-based milk
¼ cup (59 ml) canola oil, expeller pressed
1 teaspoon vanilla
1½ tablespoons maple syrup
2 tablespoons chia seeds (see Notes on page 139)
1½ cups (180 g) white whole wheat flour
1 tablespoon baking powder
1 tablespoon pumpkin pie spice
½ cup (74 g) chopped dates
¼ cup plus 2 tablespoons (85 g) chopped pumpkin seeds, shelled

1. Preheat the oven to 375° F (190°C).
2. Spray a 12-cup muffin tin with nonstick cooking spray.
3. Combine the pumpkin, plant-based milk, canola oil, vanilla, maple syrup, and chia seeds in a medium mixing bowl and mix vigorously for 2 minutes using an electric mixer or wire whisk.
4. Add the flour, baking powder, pumpkin pie spice, dates, and ¼ cup of the pumpkin seeds and mix with the mixer or a spoon until just combined, being careful not to overmix.
5. Pour the batter evenly into the prepared muffin tin and sprinkle the tops with the remaining 2 tablespoons of pumpkin seeds.
6. Bake the muffins for about 40 minutes, until brown on top and a toothpick inserted into the center of a muffin comes out clean.

note: To store the muffins in the freezer, let them cool completely, then seal them in an airtight container or bag and freeze. To serve, remove the muffins ahead of time and allow to thaw, or heat them for 30 seconds in the microwave.

variation: To make this gluten-free, substitute an all-purpose gluten-free flour blend (such as Bob's Red Mill or King Arthur Flour) for the white whole wheat flour and check that all other ingredients are gluten-free.

PER SERVING: 196 calories, 6 g protein, 24 g carbohydrate, 9 g fat, .5 g saturated fat, 4 g fiber, 9 g sugar, 15 mg sodium
STAR NUTRIENTS: riboflavin (13% DV), vitamin A (33% DV), calcium (14% DV), magnesium (12% DV), manganese (11% DV)

---

stir-fried barley with sea vegetables and peanuts

ACTIVE PREPARATION TIME: **11 minutes** • TOTAL PREPARATION TIME: **45 minutes**

You don't have to resort to potatoes, pasta, and rice for dinner every night. A whole world of whole grains awaits you! Barley, the kernel best known for beer making and barley soup, is a versatile ingredient in a variety of dishes, including pilafs and simple stir-fries. This low-glycemic grain is rich in a unique fiber called beta-glucan, which lowers blood cholesterol. Peanuts, green onions, and sea vegetables give the barley an Asian flair, making this a suitable side to dishes such as Thai Lettuce Wraps (page 240) or Savory Shiitake and White Bean Bake (page 292).

MAKES 6 SERVINGS
(about ⅔ cup each)

1 cup (200 g) uncooked pearl barley
3 cups (711 ml) water
1 teaspoon peanut oil
1 medium garlic clove, minced
½ tablespoon reduced sodium soy sauce
Dash of crushed red pepper
½ tablespoon hemp seeds
3 tablespoons coarsely chopped peanuts
¼ cup (24 g) chopped green onions, white and green parts
1 tablespoon sliced dried sea vegetables (see Note)

1. Combine the barley and water in a medium pot, cover, and cook over medium heat for about 35 to 40 minutes, until tender. Drain any remaining water. (Alternatively, cook according to manufacturer's directions in a rice cooker.)
2. Heat the peanut oil in a large skillet and add the cooked barley, garlic, soy sauce, crushed red pepper, hemp seeds, peanuts, green onions, and sea vegetables.
3. Stir-fry for about 5 minutes. Serve immediately.

note: Dried sea vegetables are increasingly available at natural food stores and conventional supermarkets, as well as Asian markets. Look for packages of sliced dried sea vegetables, such as seaweed or kelp, and experiment with them as a seasoning for dishes. Their salty taste—without the sodium—can ramp up the flavor in salads, spreads, grain dishes, Asian stir-fries and noodle dishes, and soups.

variations: You may substitute 1 cup of brown rice, quinoa, sorghum, or farro for the barley; cook according to the package instructions. (All but farro would make this dish gluten-free, with the use of gluten-free soy sauce.)

If desired, add 8 ounces (227 g) cubed firm tofu in step 2 (pressed, for best results—see page 103).

You may substitute sesame, chia, or flaxseeds for the hemp seeds.

PER SERVING: 147 calories, 5 g protein, 24 g carbohydrate, 4 g fat, .5 g saturated fat, 6 g fiber, 1 g sugar, 91 mg sodium

STAR NUTRIENTS: niacin (11% DV), thiamin (14% DV), vitamin B6 (11% DV), vitamin K (12% DV), iron (11% DV), magnesium (15% DV), manganese (36% DV), molybdenum (20% DV), phosphorus (11% DV), selenium (17% DV)

Pinto Bean and
Tofu Breakfast
Rancheros

Find the time for a truly balanced breakfast.

Pinto Bean and Tofu Breakfast Rancheros
Peanut Butter and Banana Quinoa Breakfast Bowl
Pear Buckwheat Pancakes

Skipping meals means missing out on an opportunity to fuel your body—blood, muscles, organs—with powerful nutrition. Studies consistently show that you can perform better, both mentally and physically, and maintain a healthier weight when you consume regular meals—especially breakfast. That's because eating breakfast cuts down on bad choices you may make when hunger hits you mid-morning, and it may also have some metabolism benefits. "Breaking the fast" tells your body it's not starving; thus, it's time to rev up the engine. Even if you eat the same amount of calories over an entire day, eating a larger percentage of them in the morning can help you lose weight, compared to loading up at nighttime, according to new research.

So, you can see that breakfast really is the most important meal of the day. But that doesn't mean that any old breakfast is good. One filled with refined carbs, such as sweetened and refined cold cereal, bagels, and pastries, won't help you face the day. Instead, power up on whole plant foods at breakfast every morning—even if it's as simple as oatmeal with fruit, nuts, and soy milk (see page 212). The picture-perfect breakfast combines all of the major plant food groups—whole grains, plant proteins (such as nuts, legumes, or soy), and whole fruit or vegetables (yes, that's right)—into one wholesome, satisfying meal.

Even if you're in a rush, you can start your day right with easy solutions, such as precooked whole grain porridge that you can zap in the microwave, or toasted whole grain bread with nut butter and banana slices. Get even more creative by making a veggie breakfast sandwich with sliced vegetables and greens with tahini; stir-frying vegetables, spices, and tofu into a plant-powered scramble; or feasting on a corn tortilla filled with beans and vegetables. Or throw plant-based milk, nuts or seeds, and fruit in a blender and whiz it all up for a breakfast you can sip on your morning commute (see page 287). These plant-powered breakfasts, rich in fiber and protein, will keep you satisfied until your lunch break, and they'll fuel your body with the essential vitamins, minerals, amino acids, and fats that you need to keep you at your best.

See photo
on page 134

pinto bean and tofu breakfast rancheros

ACTIVE PREPARATION TIME: 9 minutes • TOTAL PREPARATION TIME: 12 minutes

In the time it takes to go through a morning drive-through, you could feast on this satisfying dish, inspired by the huevos rancheros of Mexico, which include eggs, beans, fresh corn tortillas, and spicy salsa. My version substitutes tofu for the eggs. And who says you have to reserve this dish for breakfast? It's a tempting, easy meal for any time.

MAKES 2 SERVINGS
(1 tortilla sandwich each)

1 teaspoon extra virgin olive oil
⅓ cup (77 g) canned vegetarian refried pinto beans
Four 6-inch (15 cm) corn tortillas
⅓ cup (95 g) finely diced extra firm tofu (pressed, for best results—see page 103)
2 tablespoons finely chopped black olives
2 tablespoons prepared Fresh Guacamole with Tomatoes and Serrano Chiles (page 205)
2 tablespoons prepared salsa
2 tablespoons chopped green onions, green parts only
Plant-based sour cream, optional (see Note on page 344)

1. Heat ½ teaspoon of the olive oil in a small skillet over medium heat.
2. Spread 3 tablespoons of refried beans onto a tortilla.
3. Place the tortilla in the skillet with the bean side up. Sprinkle with 3 tablespoons of the tofu and 1 tablespoon of the black olives. Place another tortilla on top of the bean mixture and press with a spatula. Cook for 2 to 3 minutes, until golden.
4. Turn and cook the other side for 2 to 3 minutes, until golden.
5. Remove from the heat and place on a serving dish. Repeat this process to prepare the second bean-tofu tortilla.
6. Garnish each tortilla sandwich with guacamole, salsa, green onions, and plant-based sour cream, if desired.

variation: Substitute refried black beans or mashed lentils for the pinto beans; substitute small flavored whole grain tortillas for corn tortillas.

PER SERVING: 249 calories, 9 g protein, 32 g carbohydrate, 10 g fat, 1 g saturated fat, 6 g fiber, 2 g sugar, 309 mg sodium
STAR NUTRIENTS: calcium (10% DV), iron (10% DV), magnesium (14% DV)

peanut butter and banana quinoa breakfast bowl

ACTIVE PREPARATION TIME: **9 minutes** • TOTAL PREPARATION TIME: **22 minutes**

Who says you can't eat quinoa at breakfast? A number of whole grains make excellent breakfast porridges. The classic American pairing of peanuts and bananas elevates this cereal into star status among the whole family—from the youngest to the oldest. Make a whole pot and microwave the leftovers later for the next morning.

MAKES 4 SERVINGS
(generous ½ cup quinoa each, plus toppings)

1 cup (170 g) uncooked quinoa
2 cups (474 ml) water
1 teaspoon vanilla extract
2 tablespoons unsalted creamy or crunchy peanut butter
2 medium ripe bananas, sliced
¼ cup (23 g) unsweetened shredded coconut
2 tablespoons chopped peanuts
Plant-based milk, optional

1. Place the quinoa and water in a medium pot, cover, and bring to a boil over medium-high heat. Reduce heat to medium and cook for 10 to 12 minutes, until tender.
2. Stir in the vanilla and peanut butter and divide the quinoa among four cereal bowls.
3. Top with the bananas, coconut, and peanuts. Serve with plant-based milk, if desired.

note: If you are going to serve this porridge later, do not add the bananas, coconut, and peanuts until after reheating, to avoid discoloration and sogginess.

variation: Replace the peanuts and peanut butter with sunflower seeds and sunflower seed butter or almonds and almond butter.

PER SERVING: 289 calories, 10 g protein, 42 g carbohydrate, 10.5 g fat, 3 g saturated fat, 6 g fiber, 7 g sugar, 9 mg sodium
STAR NUTRIENTS: folate (25% DV), niacin (14% DV), riboflavin (11% DV), thiamin (13% DV), vitamin B6 (23% DV), vitamin E (10% DV), copper (22% DV), iron (13% DV), magnesium (30% DV), manganese (69% DV), phosphorus (27% DV), potassium (15% DV), zinc (13% DV)

pear buckwheat pancakes

ACTIVE PREPARATION TIME: **15 minutes** • TOTAL PREPARATION TIME: **30 minutes**

Start your day right with a balance of whole grains, fruit, and protein. The pseudo cereal grain buckwheat (it's actually a seed in the sorrel and rhubarb family!) has a wild, nutty flavor that perfectly accents baked goods, such as hearty pancakes. In this whole grain pancake recipe, pear sauce adds natural sweetness to the mix, and almonds add crunch. It's a great start for a relaxed Saturday, or a school-day breakfast for your child.

MAKES 8 SERVINGS
(1 pancake each)

½ cup (122 g) pear sauce (see Notes)
1 tablespoon chia seeds (see Notes)
1 cup (237 ml) unsweetened plain plant-based milk
2 tablespoons canola oil, expeller pressed
2 tablespoons maple syrup
1 teaspoon cinnamon
1 tablespoon baking powder
1 cup (120 g) whole wheat flour (white whole wheat or whole
   wheat pastry flour, if desired)
½ cup (60 g) buckwheat flour
⅓ cup (31 g) finely chopped almonds
Nonstick cooking spray

1. Mix together the pear sauce, chia seeds, plant-based milk, canola oil, and maple syrup and beat vigorously with a whisk or electric mixer for 2 minutes.

2. Add the cinnamon, baking powder, whole wheat flour, buckwheat flour, and almonds. Combine well, but do not overstir.

3. Heat a pancake griddle or large cast-iron skillet over medium heat. Spray with nonstick cooking spray. Add ¼ cup of batter to the pan, and spread with a spatula to make a thin pancake. Cook (in batches of four each) for about 3 minutes on each side, until golden brown and cooked through.

4. Repeat for a total of 8 pancakes. Serve immediately.

notes: To make your own pear sauce, see page 343.

Chia seeds, when combined with liquid, create a gel that can help provide some of the binding power that eggs lend to dishes.

variations: You may substitute applesauce for the pear sauce, and pecans, walnuts, or hazelnuts for the almonds. For a gluten-free version, substitute ⅔ cup gluten-free flour blend (such as Bob's Red Mill or King Arthur Flour) for the whole wheat flour in step 2, and check that all other ingredients are gluten-free.

PER SERVING: 214 calories, 6 g protein, 33 g carbohydrate, 8 g fat, 1 g saturated fat, 5 g fiber, 7 g sugar, 199 mg sodium

STAR NUTRIENTS: riboflavin (11% DV), thiamin (12% DV), vitamin C (13% DV), vitamin E (11% DV), calcium (28% DV), iron (10% DV), magnesium (12% DV), manganese (22% DV), phosphorus (12% DV)

Curried Tofu
Papaya Wraps

Eat well on the run.

Bombay Carrot, Beet, and Bulgur Salad
Curried Tofu Papaya Wraps

When you're cooking plant-powered meals from scratch—calling upon wholesome ingredients, such as whole grains, lentils, and seasonal vegetables in healthful combinations—it's easy to meet your goals for health. But it's much harder when you're eating on the run, especially if you rely on fast-food drive-throughs and casual eateries. A recent study found that adults' fast-food meals contained an average of 836 calories, 41 percent of their total average calorie needs for the entire day. And chain restaurants faired even worse: a Tufts University study found that the average calorie content of these meals totaled 1,327—66 percent of the total calorie requirement for the day.

Thankfully, some restaurants are now doing a better job with their plant-based menu options. Casual restaurants serve up vegan foods, like quinoa kale salad or tofu curry with brown rice. Even some quick-service restaurants offer creative fare, such as brown rice chickpea salad or veggie burgers on whole grain buns. However, these choices pale in comparison to the plant-powered "fast food" meals you can make for yourself, often inexpensively and time-effectively.

In the winter, cook up a one-dish stew and pack the leftovers in a micro-wavable container in an insulated lunch bag for the next day in the office. In the summer, you can switch to a vegetable-grain salad, accompanied with a small bag of nuts for a protein boost. Any time of year, get creative with a tofu-vegetable wrap, grilled veggie sandwich, or bean and avocado burrito.

And don't stop with work lunches: pack up goodies for picnics in the park, hikes, or beach days. When you're traveling—whether on the road or by plane—pack smart! Don't let poor plant-food availability derail your best intentions for health. Spread nut or seed butter on whole grain bread with fruit spread and add an apple for a nonperishable meal that will satisfy. If you have access to transportation, stop by a natural food store, which often offers amazing takeout choices, such as creative entrée salads brimming with grains, greens, and legumes. And if you're really stuck—in an airport or a highway—choose hummus and veggie sticks, green salads, whole pieces of fruit, packs of nuts or seeds, and dried fruit.

bombay carrot, beet, and bulgur salad

ACTIVE PREPARATION TIME: **17 minutes** • TOTAL PREPARATION TIME: **40 minutes**

You can avoid fast-food pitfalls by packing your own lunch. Try creating this colorful, crunchy salad the night before, and pack it into a container the next day. Pair it with a protein-rich food (baked tofu slices, plant-based yogurt, flatbread with sunflower seed butter) and a piece of fruit and you're good to go. You'll also be the envy of the break room!

MAKES 8 SERVINGS
(about ¾ cup each)

1½ cups (273 g) cooked bulgur wheat, cooled
8 ounces (232 g) cubed cooked beets (see Notes)
1½ cups (165 g) shredded carrots
2 tablespoons (20 g) finely diced white onion
⅓ cup (55 g) raisins
¼ cup (15 g) chopped cilantro or parsley
2 tablespoons orange juice
1 tablespoon extra virgin olive oil
¼ teaspoon crushed red pepper, or to taste
½ teaspoon garam masala (see Notes)
¼ teaspoon turmeric
Pinch of sea salt, optional
¼ cup (36 g) coarsely chopped peanuts

1. Toss together the bulgur wheat, beets, carrots, onion, raisins, and cilantro.
2. In a small dish, make the dressing by whisking together the orange juice, olive oil, crushed red pepper, garam masala, and turmeric.
3. Add the dressing to the salad and toss well to coat. Taste and add a pinch of sea salt, if desired.
4. Garnish with the peanuts immediately before serving.

notes: If you're in a rush, use precooked beets (refrigerated or canned) and preshredded carrots, widely available in most supermarkets.

Garam masala is an Indian spice blend that may be found in many gourmet or ethnic food stores, as well as online.

If you're planning on storing leftovers or serving this the following day, reserve the peanuts for adding at the last minute.

variations: For a gluten-free alternative, substitute cooked brown rice for the bulgur wheat in step 1.

PER SERVING: 113 calories, 3 g protein, 18 g carbohydrate, 4 g fat, .5 g saturated fat, 3 g fiber, 7 g sugar, 41 mg sodium
STAR NUTRIENTS: folate (11% DV), vitamin A (70% DV), vitamin C (16% DV), manganese (19% DV)

See photo
on page 140

curried tofu papaya wraps

ACTIVE PREPARATION TIME: **18 minutes** • TOTAL PREPARATION TIME: **48 minutes**
(including chilling time)

Now this is what I call healthy, delicious eating on the run! Filled with a colorful, flavorful tofu, papaya, and coconut filling, this wrap is a delicious treat as an appetizer or for lunch. Stock up on powerful nutrients, such as beta-carotene, vitamin C, fiber, and protein in this meal-in-one.

MAKES 6 SERVINGS
(one 9-inch wrap each)

½ cup (119 g) canned light coconut milk (well mixed before
measured)
1½ teaspoons Thai red curry paste
½ teaspoon minced fresh ginger
1 medium garlic clove, minced
½ teaspoon turmeric
½ teaspoon reduced sodium soy sauce
Pinch of cayenne pepper (see Notes)
One 12-ounce (340 g) package extra firm tofu, drained and
cubed (pressed, for best results—see page 103)
1 medium papaya, peeled and diced
½ cup (48 g) chopped green onions, white and green parts
¼ cup (15 g) chopped fresh cilantro
Pinch of sea salt, optional
Six 9-inch (23 cm) whole grain tortillas or wraps
3 cups (102 g) fresh watercress, or baby salad greens, if
unavailable

1. Mix together the coconut milk, curry paste, ginger, garlic, turmeric, soy sauce, and cayenne in a mixing bowl until smooth.
2. Fold in the tofu, papaya, green onions, and cilantro. Taste and season with sea salt, if desired. Refrigerate for 30 minutes (or overnight, if desired).
3. Place one tortilla on a cutting board. Spread ½ cup of the tofu mixture down the center of the tortilla in a row. Top with ½ cup of the watercress.
4. Fold the right side of the tortilla over the center and start to wrap tightly, pressing in as you wrap. Place the wrap on a serving dish seam side down.
5. Serve as a whole wrap for an individual meal (cut in half for easier eating), or slice into thin pinwheels for an appetizer.

notes: Adjust the spiciness of the wraps by increasing the cayenne pepper.

Store the curried tofu wraps in plastic wrap or in an airtight container as a perfect lunch to go.

If you won't be consuming all of the wraps at one time, reserve the filling in an airtight container in the refrigerator and prepare the wraps no more than 4 hours before serving time to prevent the greens from wilting and the wrap from getting soggy.

variation: If papaya is not available, substitute 1 large mango or 2 large peaches.

PER SERVING: 213 calories, 10 g protein, 32 g carbohydrate, 5 g fat, 1.5 g saturated fat, 5 g fiber, 6 g sugar, 256 mg sodium
STAR NUTRIENTS: folate (10% DV), niacin (11% DV), thiamin (17% DV), vitamin A (30% DV), vitamin C (80% DV), calcium (19% DV), iron (14% DV), magnesium (10% DV), phosphorus (21% DV), zinc (10% DV)

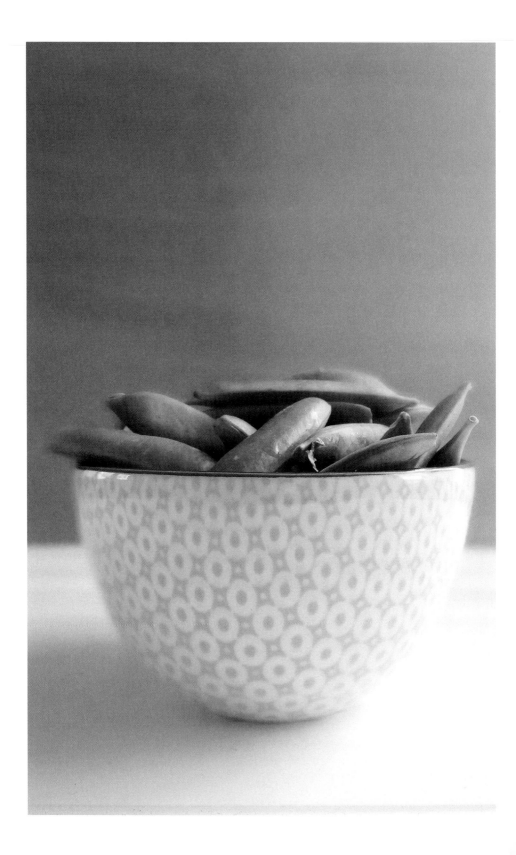

Snack right!

Edamame Hummus
Crispy Ginger-Amaranth Cookies

Maybe when you were a kid your mom told you to stay out of the kitchen so you wouldn't "spoil your appetite." But busy modern lifestyles—with dual-income households, an increase in after-hours activities, such as sports or evening classes, and longer work commutes—have made snacking more popular than ever. Now, many of us purposefully snack to fuel our mental or athletic performances, recover from exercise, and quell hunger pains. Partly because of this changed attitude to snacking, the number of snacks we consume has doubled over the past three decades. As we hunker over laptops, fit more activities into our schedules, and spend more time on the road, research shows that we are spending less time at the dinner table and more time eating mini-meals elsewhere.

While you don't *have* to snack for optimal health, it can help you feel more satisfied, less hungry, and less likely to make poor eating choices later. If you find that you struggle with hunger or concentration mid-meal, you are likely the perfect candidate for a mid-meal snack. However, if your snacks are nothing but a low-nutrient treat to satisfy a sweet tooth or salt craving, then you are missing out on an opportunity to fit important nutrients into your day.

Americans fall short on fiber, potassium, calcium, and vitamin D; and we don't meet our needs for fruits and vegetables, which power our bodies with potent antioxidant and anti-inflammatory compounds. If snacking takes up a part of your daily diet, than those food choices need to contribute these nutrients to your daily diet that support optimal health. And in order to gain a sense of fullness, your snack should provide a bit of protein, healthy fats, and carbs. But that doesn't mean you have to hunker up to a 500-calorie snack! Unless you're an athlete, just a small 100- to 150-calorie snack will suffice. A handful of nuts and raisins, a homemade nutrition bar (see page 206), or a carton of soy yogurt are perfect examples.

Skip the empty food choices, such as sugary granola bars, cookies, chips, and refined crackers. Let snacks provide an opportunity to fit in important servings of legumes, nuts, seeds, fruits, and veggies every day.

edamame hummus

ACTIVE PREPARATION TIME: **8 minutes** • TOTAL PREPARATION TIME: **8 minutes**

I believe that every plant-powered kitchen should have a container of homemade hummus in the refrigerator. It's a great snack with whole grain pita and fresh veggies, as well as a nutrient-rich spread for sandwiches, wraps, and veggie burgers. The "clean" ingredients list of homemade hummus—which can be whizzed up in minutes—is much more wholesome than you'll find in many store-bought versions. A serving of this edamame hummus rakes in 5 grams of protein!

MAKES 10 SERVINGS
(about ¼ cup each)

One 15-ounce (425 g) can chickpeas, drained (liquid reserved)
2 medium garlic cloves, minced
Juice of 1 medium lemon
2 tablespoons tahini
2 teaspoons extra virgin olive oil
½ teaspoon smoked paprika
1 cup (150 g) shelled cooked edamame, thawed and drained if frozen
¼ cup (15 g) chopped fresh parsley
Pinch of sea salt, optional

1. Place the chickpeas, garlic, lemon juice, tahini, olive oil, paprika, edamame, and parsley in a blender.
2. Add ⅓ cup of the reserved chickpea liquid. Process the mixture until smooth, scraping down the sides as needed. Add additional reserved liquid as needed to make a smooth, thick hummus. Taste and season with a pinch of sea salt, if desired.
3. Chill until serving time. Serve cold or at room temperature with whole wheat pita segments and fresh veggies, or on sandwiches.

note: This recipe stores well in an airtight container in the refrigerator for up to 3 days.

variations: Substitute canned white beans for the chickpeas.

PER SERVING: 86 calories, 5 g protein, 9 g carbohydrate, 4 g fat, .5 g saturated fat, 3 g fiber, 3 g sugar, 122 mg sodium

STAR NUTRIENTS: folate (16% DV), vitamin B6 (12% DV), vitamin C (19% DV), vitamin K (31% DV), manganese (19% DV)

---

crispy ginger-amaranth cookies

ACTIVE PREPARATION TIME: **13 minutes** • TOTAL PREPARATION TIME: **30 minutes**

One of the simple pleasures of life is baking—the art of folding together ingredients to create tasty, fragrant baked goods, such as cookies. And these crispy, gingery cookies are an indulgence you can feel good about! They call upon a whole grain staple of the ancient Aztecs—amaranth, a versatile grain traditionally used in porridges. When popped—as it is in this recipe—amaranth offers a nutty, crunchy bite.

MAKES 20 SERVINGS
(1 cookie each)

Nonstick cooking spray
¼ cup (48 g) uncooked amaranth
1½ cups (180 g) amaranth flour
1 teaspoon ground ginger
1½ teaspoons baking powder
½ cup (66 g) chopped macadamia nuts
¼ cup (57 g) soft dairy-free margarine (see Notes on page 223)
½ cup (74 g) finely chopped dates
¼ cup (84 g) molasses
¼ cup (84 g) agave nectar

1. Preheat the oven to 350°F (180°C). Spray a baking sheet with nonstick cooking spray.
2. Place a small pot over medium heat for 1 minute. Add the amaranth and heat, stirring, for about 6 minutes, allowing the grains to toast and pop.
3. In a medium mixing bowl, stir together the popped amaranth, amaranth flour, ginger, baking powder, and macadamia nuts.
4. Stir in the margarine, dates, molasses, and agave until smooth.
5. Drop cookies by the heaping tablespoonful onto the prepared baking sheet.
6. Bake for 18 to 20 minutes, until cooked through and golden.

notes: These cookies may be frozen for up to one month.

This recipe is gluten-free as long as you check that all ingredients—particularly the amaranth, amaranth flour, and baking powder—are gluten-free.

variation: Substitute walnuts, pecans, hazelnuts, or sunflower seeds for the macadamia nuts.

PER SERVING: 134 calories, 3 g protein, 21 g carbohydrate, 5 g fat, 1 g saturated fat, 2 g fiber, 9 g sugar, 18 mg sodium
STAR NUTRIENTS: magnesium (15% DV), manganese (16% DV)

Yellow Squash Stuffed
with Saffron Rye Berries

Spend some time cooking every day—
and enjoy it.

Sun-Dried Tomato and Olive Chickpea Focaccia
Yellow Squash Stuffed with Saffron Rye Berries
Vegetable Ribbon Salad with Lime Vinaigrette

❦

What am I going to make for dinner? We often ask ourselves that at the end of the day—perhaps with a groan. Many of us dread this daily obligation, especially when tired, hungry, and short on inspiration.

Yet, in many cultures, cooking symbolizes good fortune—the gift of plenty. Throughout history, the time-honored tradition of taking raw ingredients and turning them into delicious meals that can sustain a family has been regarded as one of the most important tasks of life.

Indeed, having enough food to cook is worthy of celebration. Throughout our frail human story, one of our biggest challenges was simply having enough nutritious food in order to survive. In today's society of surplus calories, oversize Styrofoam takeout trays, and mega-bags of snack foods, we've lost sight of being thankful for an ample food supply.

In the past, children learned to cook from their parents or at school. Now, with cooking classes banished from standard school curricula, and few parents making the time to teach (or even cook themselves), we are in our second generation of non-cooks. Seven percent of Americans don't cook at all, and one in five says that they do not enjoy it.

I implore you to think about cooking with fresh eyes. Let this time of the day be your meditation and time for gratitude as you chop celery for a soup, dice onions to sauté, and wash tender leaves of lettuce for a salad; let the day's stress fall off your shoulders like rain. Take a deep breath as you toast cumin in olive oil or mince garlic for a marinade, and let the aromas lift your spirits and take you away. Then sit down to eat the meal you've prepared. Whether you share it with friends and family or enjoy it on your own, let food be an expression of love.

sun-dried tomato and olive chickpea focaccia

ACTIVE PREPARATION TIME: 17 minutes • TOTAL PREPARATION TIME: 1 hour 30 minutes

When you have some extra time—say, on a relaxed weekend—indulge your creative side and try your hand at homemade bread. Let the amazing flavors and aromas be your reward! This easy focaccia—a traditional flat Italian bread tenderized with olive oil and topped with herbs—is based on nutritious chickpea and/or fava bean flours. Whip up the dough, let it rise, stud it with garlic, herbs, sun-dried tomatoes, and olives, and you've got a flavorful accompaniment for a soup, such as Tomato Barley Soup (page 263), or salad, like Apple and Fennel Salad with Arugula (page 192). Alternatively, set out a platter of this focaccia at a party and watch it disappear!

MAKES 12 SERVINGS
(1 slice each)

Focaccia Dough
1 cup (120 g) chickpea or fava bean flour (see Notes)
1½ cups (180 g) whole wheat pastry flour
1 package (2½ teaspoons) instant yeast
1 teaspoon honey or agave nectar
1¼ cups (296 ml) lukewarm water
1 teaspoon reserved olive oil from sun-dried tomatoes (see below)
Pinch of kosher salt, optional
Nonstick cooking spray

Topping
Half of an 8-ounce (227 g) jar sun-dried tomatoes in olive oil, drained (oil reserved)
16 Italian olives (such as Ligurian, Ponentine, or Lugano; see Notes)
2 medium garlic cloves, finely chopped
⅓ cup (8 g) sliced fresh basil leaves
Freshly ground black pepper

1. To make the focaccia dough, combine the chickpea flour, whole wheat pastry flour, yeast, honey, and water in a medium mixing bowl. Add one teaspoon of the olive oil from the jar of sun-dried tomatoes and the pinch of salt, if desired. Using an electric mixer, blend well for 5 minutes to make a soft, sticky dough. Cover the bowl with a towel and place in a warm place for 1 hour to rise.

2. Preheat the oven to 400°F (205°C). Spray a large baking sheet with nonstick cooking spray and spread the dough out on it into a thin layer, about 9 by 13 inches large.

3. Press the sun-dried tomatoes and olives into the dough. Sprinkle evenly with the garlic, basil, and black pepper to taste.
4. Bake for 18 to 20 minutes, until cooked through and golden.
5. Slice into 12 rectangular pieces. Serve warm.

notes: You can find chickpea or fava bean flour in natural food stores, the gluten-free aisle of large supermarkets, or online. You can also try a garbanzo-fava blend (sometimes known as garfava flour).

If you can't find Italian olives, substitute kalamata or Spanish olives.

Store leftovers in an airtight container in the refrigerator for up to 3 days and reheat before serving.

variations: Add additional toppings, such as plant-based cheese, canned white beans (drained, no salt added), or pine nuts for a hearty appetizer or entrée. To make this bread gluten-free, substitute a gluten-free flour blend (such as Bob's Red Mill or King Arthur Flour) for the whole wheat pastry flour, and increase baking time to 25 to 30 minutes.

PER SERVING: 131 calories, 5 g protein, 21 g carbohydrate, 3 g fat, 0 g saturated fat, 4 g fiber, 2 g sugar, 69 mg sodium
STAR NUTRIENTS: folate (12% DV), thiamin (10% DV), vitamin C (24% DV), iron (10% DV), manganese (12% DV)

See photo
on page 152

yellow squash stuffed with saffron rye berries

ACTIVE PREPARATION TIME: 20 minutes • TOTAL PREPARATION TIME: 1 hour 15 minutes

Inventive ways to cook with plants make spending time in the kitchen fresh and fun. One of my favorite techniques is stuffing vegetables. Veggies with tender, edible skins, like squash and bell peppers, are just begging to be stuffed with flavorful ingredients! The extra thought and presentation of this dish makes it a feast for the eyes, as well as the body and soul. Savory rye berries with a subtle scent of saffron form the crunchy, nutritious filling in these sunny squash halves. This stuffed squash is elegant enough to serve at a special dinner yet simple enough to put on the menu any night of the week. Pair it with a bean dish, such as Lentils with Wild Mushrooms and Broccoli Rabe (page 230).

MAKES 4 SERVINGS
(½ squash each)

....

¼ cup (42 g) uncooked rye berries
2 cups (474 ml) water
1 teaspoon reduced sodium vegetable broth base
10 saffron threads, crushed
2 medium (196 g each, about 7 inches long) yellow summer
    squash (e.g., straightneck; see Notes)
1 teaspoon extra virgin olive oil
½ small (35 g) yellow onion, finely diced
½ medium (60 g) green bell pepper, finely diced
½ cup (35 g) finely chopped mushrooms
1 medium garlic clove, minced
Pinch of freshly ground black pepper
2 tablespoons minced fresh parsley, plus more for garnish,
    optional
¼ cup (29 g) finely chopped hazelnuts, plus more for garnish,
    optional

1. Place the rye berries in a small pot with the water and broth base. Cover with a lid and cook over medium heat for 30 minutes, stirring occasionally. Add the saffron, cover, and cook for an additional 10 minutes, stirring occasionally. Replace water lost to evaporation as needed to prevent burning. When finished, drain any leftover liquid and set the rye berries aside.

2. Meanwhile, slice the squash horizontally in half and scoop out their interiors (see Notes), leaving about one inch of flesh around the peel. Place in a small baking dish, hollow side up.

3. Preheat the oven to 350°F (180°C).

4. Heat the olive oil in a small sauté pan or skillet over medium heat. Add the onion and cook for 2 minutes. Add the bell pepper, mushrooms, and garlic and sauté for an additional 4 minutes.

5. Add the black pepper, parsley, hazelnuts, and cooked rye berries to the vegetable mixture and mix well.

6. Mound the rye berries–vegetable filling into the cavity of each summer squash (approximately ¼ cup for each squash). Add ½ inch of water to the bottom of the baking dish.

7. Cover the baking dish with foil and bake for 30 minutes.

8. Uncover and bake for an additional 10 minutes, until the filling is browned and the squash is tender. If desired, garnish with additional parsley and chopped hazelnuts before serving.

notes: Try to select smooth, straight yellow squash for this recipe, so that they are easy to fill and lie flat in the baking dish.

Don't discard the unused squash pulp; use it in another dish, such as Shanghai Stir-Fry with Forbidden Rice (page 2).

variations: Substitute uncooked ¼ cup quinoa (a gluten-free alternative) for the rye berries, and cook with 1 cup water for 20 minutes, according to directions in step 1.

Substitute medium zucchinis or large bell peppers for the yellow squash.

PER SERVING: 185 calories, 7 g protein, 20 g carbohydrate, 11 g fat, 1 g saturated fat, 6 g fiber, 6 g sugar, 303 mg sodium
STAR NUTRIENTS: folate (16% DV), niacin (10% DV), riboflavin (16% DV), thiamin (12% DV), vitamin A (11% DV), vitamin B6 (23% DV), vitamin C (83% DV), vitamin E (14% DV), vitamin K (46% DV), copper (13% DV), iron (11% DV), magnesium (15% DV), manganese (34% DV), molybdenum (17% DV), potassium (19% DV)

vegetable ribbon salad with lime vinaigrette

ACTIVE PREPARATION TIME: **18 minutes** • TOTAL PREPARATION TIME: **18 minutes**

Learn some new plant-powered culinary techniques as you make time for your daily meditation in the kitchen. For example, lovely thin ribbons of tender garden-fresh produce, such as the asparagus, summer squash, and carrots in this salad, can create a simple yet stunning dish. Tossed with a delicate vinaigrette, this vegetable ribbon salad makes a beautiful contribution to any meal. If you're really crafty, purchase a handheld mandoline, which creates perfect thin ribbons; however, you can rely on your trusty vegetable peeler to get the job done as well. The peels are not removed, as they add lovely color—and nutrition—to the ribbons.

MAKES 4 SERVINGS
(about 1 cup each)

1 small Persian cucumber (see Notes)
1 small yellow summer squash (e.g., straightneck)
1 small zucchini
1 medium carrot
4 large spears asparagus
2 medium radishes
½ tablespoon extra virgin olive oil
1 teaspoon lime juice
½ teaspoon lime zest
½ teaspoon honey or agave nectar
¼ teaspoon dry mustard
Pinch of white pepper
2 tablespoons chopped fresh chives
1½ teaspoons sesame seeds

1. Without peeling, clean and trim the cucumber, squash, zucchini, carrot, asparagus, and radishes (see Notes), then use a vegetable peeler or mandoline to create long, thin ribbons.

2. Place vegetable ribbons on a plate covered with paper towels to remove excess liquid; after a few minutes, transfer them to a salad bowl.

3. In a small dish, make the vinaigrette by whisking together the olive oil, lime juice, lime zest, honey, mustard, and white pepper.

4. Add the vinaigrette to the ribbons and toss gently with a fork, just to distribute it well.

5. Sprinkle with the chives and sesame seeds and serve immediately.

notes: Petite, sweet, and tender Persian cucumbers are perfect for a ribbon salad. If you can't find these, substitute half of a small English cucumber.

The seedy inner cores of the summer squash and zucchini, as well as any centers of the other vegetables you find difficult to peel into ribbons, may be saved and added to a soup or stir-fry later. Make this recipe immediately before serving and cut it in half if you're planning a meal for two; this delicate salad does not store well.

PER SERVING: 70 calories, 2 g protein, 7 g carbohydrate, 4 g fat, .5 g saturated fat, 2 g fiber, 4 g sugar, 30 mg sodium

STAR NUTRIENTS: folate (11% DV), vitamin A (56% DV), vitamin C (29% DV), manganese (11% DV), potassium (10% DV)

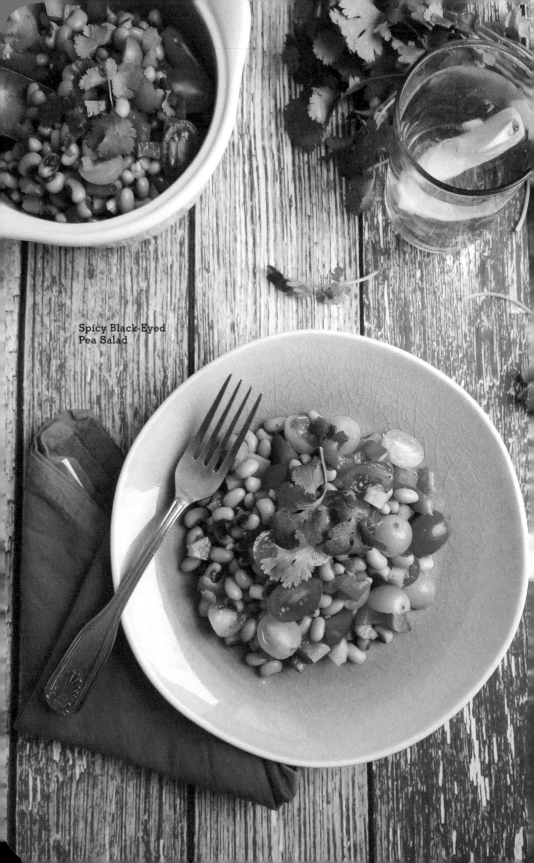

Spicy Black-Eyed
Pea Salad

Put real foods first.

Spicy Black-Eyed Pea Salad
Buckwheat Tabbouleh
Teff Porridge with Dates, Figs, and Pistachios

It seems like everyone's popping supplement pills these days. In fact, we're spending $32 billion per year on dietary supplements, such as vitamins, minerals, and antioxidants. Indeed, the most important thing you can do for your health is to fuel your body with good nutrition—researchers now list an unhealthful diet as the number one cause for poor health and early death. If you fill up on calorie-laden, nutrition-poor foods such as snack foods, cookies, and sugary beverages, you'll be missing out on all of the nutrients your body needs to keep humming at optimal function. But if you plan well, make every bite count, and pack your diet with whole plant foods—whole grains, legumes, fruits, vegetables, seeds, and nuts—you won't need to rely on supplements.

In fact, the latest studies indicate you don't gain the same health benefits from eating nutrients in isolation—dietary supplements—as you do from eating them in foods. It appears that nutrients such as omega-3s, calcium, beta-carotene, antioxidants, and even those in multivitamins work better in the whole food, where they exist side by side with hundreds of other nutrients and compounds. It's also very difficult to get too much of a nutrient from food, while it's easy to overdo it and push nutrients out of balance when you swallow a capsule.

However, while an entirely plant-based diet is very healthful, a few nutrients are challenging to get. The hardest is vitamin B12, found only in animal foods. While you can get vitamin B12 in some nutritional yeasts and fortified foods, this nutrient is so vital to your health that I recommend you take a supplement every day if you avoid all animal foods, including dairy and eggs. The vitamin B12 RDA for adults ages fourteen and up is 2.4 micrograms per day. For information on calcium, vitamin D, and omega-3s, check out page 279.

See photo
on page 160

spicy black-eyed pea salad

ACTIVE PREPARATION TIME: 16 minutes • TOTAL PREPARATION TIME: 1 hour
(not including soaking time)

When you focus on whole plant foods, such as legumes—packed with dozens of essential vitamins and minerals—you don't need to worry about popping supplement pills. Unlike a pill, plant foods provide dozens of nutrients in balance and synergy; the nutrients work together to promote good health. The "lucky" black-eyed pea is the star of this flavorful, Southern-inspired salad. Rich in protein, it's a great entrée salad that can be the center of your plate, and tucked away in a lunch box the next day. Serve it with Grits Smothered with Mustard Greens (page 246) for a comforting—and nutritious—meal made in heaven.

MAKES 8 SERVINGS
(about ¾ cup each)

2 cups (410 g) dried black-eyed peas (see Note)
4 cups (948 ml) water, plus more for soaking
1 teaspoon reduced sodium vegetable broth base
2 medium garlic cloves, minced
1½ cups (224 g) cherry tomatoes (yellow and red), halved
½ cup (51 g) diced celery
½ medium bell pepper (red, yellow, or green), diced
1 small jalapeño pepper, finely diced
4 green onions, white and green parts, sliced
¼ cup (15 g) chopped parsley or cilantro
1 tablespoon extra virgin olive oil
Juice of ½ lemon
½ teaspoon chili powder
½ teaspoon Cajun seasoning blend (see page 345), or to taste
½ teaspoon agave nectar or honey
Pinch of sea salt, optional

1. Place the dried black-eyed peas in a bowl, cover with water, and soak overnight.
2. Drain off the water and place the black-eyed peas in a pot with the 4 cups of fresh water, vegetable broth base, and half of the garlic. Cover, bring to a boil over medium-high heat, and reduce the heat to medium and cook for 40 to 45 minutes, until tender yet firm. Drain any leftover liquid and let the peas cool. (If using canned or precooked black-eyed peas, skip this step, but add the garlic to the salad in step 3.)
3. Combine the cooled black-eyed peas, tomatoes, celery, bell pepper, jalapeño, green onions, and parsley in a large mixing bowl and mix well.

4. In a small dish, whisk together the olive oil, lemon juice, the remaining garlic, chili powder, Cajun seasoning, agave, and a pinch of sea salt, if desired. Pour over the black-eyed pea mixture and toss well.

5. Chill for about 30 minutes, until serving time.

note: Instead of dried beans, you may use 4½ cups precooked or canned black-eyed peas, no salt added, rinsed and drained (about two and a half 15-ounce/425 g cans).

variations: Substitute black beans, white beans, or garbanzo beans for the black-eyed peas.

PER SERVING: 135 calories, 7 g protein, 22 g carbohydrate, 3 g fat, 6 g fiber, 3 g sugar, 0 g saturated fat, 80 mg sodium

STAR NUTRIENTS: folate (10% DV), riboflavin (10% DV), thiamin (67% DV), vitamin A (14% DV), vitamin C (38% DV), vitamin K (45% DV), iron (13% DV), magnesium (18% DV), phosphorus (13% DV), potassium (11% DV), zinc (13% DV)

---

buckwheat tabbouleh

ACTIVE PREPARATION TIME: 21 minutes • TOTAL PREPARATION TIME: 30 minutes

Who needs to pop pills when you can feast on nutrient-rich foods simply packed with health-promoting power? Grain- and vegetable-based salads offer a unique opportunity to power your diet with vitamins, minerals, phyto-chemicals, and more. I swapped the bulgur found in traditional tabbouleh recipes for buckwheat, which provides a grassy, nutty tone to this salad. Rich in parsley and mint flavors, this salad is the perfect accompaniment for Middle Eastern foods, such as roasted vegetables, whole wheat pita, hum-mus, and Mediterranean Eggplant and Artichoke Lasagna (page 94).

MAKES 10 SERVINGS
(about 1 scant cup each)

1 cup (170 g) uncooked buckwheat
2 cups (474 ml) water
2 medium garlic cloves
4 cups (240 g) chopped fresh parsley, loosely packed
½ cup (12 g) mint leaves, loosely packed
5 green onions, white and green parts, finely diced
3 small Persian cucumbers, with peels, finely diced
2 medium tomatoes, finely diced
2 tablespoons extra virgin olive oil
Juice of 2 medium lemons
¼ teaspoon freshly ground black pepper
Pinch of sea salt, optional

1. Place the buckwheat in a small pot with the water. Cover and bring to a boil over medium-high heat. Reduce the heat to medium and cook for 15 minutes on medium heat, stirring occasionally.
2. Drain any remaining liquid and transfer the cooked buckwheat to a large mixing bowl and refrigerate to cool.
3. Place the garlic, parsley, and mint in a food processor. Process until only finely chopped (do not liquefy), or chop by hand, very finely. Pour into the bowl with buckwheat.
4. Add the green onions, cucumbers, and tomatoes, and mix well.
5. Mix the olive oil, lemon juice, black pepper, and sea salt, if desired, in a small dish. Add to the buckwheat mixture and toss.

variation: Substitute another cooked whole grain (or combination of grains) for the buckwheat, such as cooked bulgur, wheat berries, quinoa, rye berries, or farro. Note that buckwheat is gluten-free, whereas all of these options, except for quinoa, are not.

PER SERVING: 108 calories, 3 g protein, 18 g carbohydrate, 4 g fat, .5 g saturated fat, 4 g fiber, 2 g sugar, 22 mg sodium
STAR NUTRIENTS: folate (16% DV), vitamin A (49% DV), vitamin C (72% DV), vitamin K (536% DV), copper (11% DV), iron (13% DV), magnesium (15% DV), manganese (21% DV), potassium (10% DV)

teff porridge with dates, figs, and pistachios

ACTIVE PREPARATION TIME: **10 minutes** • TOTAL PREPARATION TIME: **22 minutes**

Mainstream breakfast cereals may be fortified with added vitamins, but they're usually also highly processed. If you put whole grains on your breakfast menu, you'll gain the benefits of the whole grain—fiber, vitamins, minerals, phytochemicals, and all. Teff is a life-giving whole grain foodstuff in its native land of Ethiopia, where it evolved to grow in drought-ridden soils over the centuries—it's believed to date back as far as 4000 BC. These tiny black seeds are rich in not only fiber, but also iron, protein, and calcium. This wholesome, rustic breakfast porridge, flavored with dried figs, dates, and pistachios, takes me on a journey to this part of the world every time I sit down to eat it.

MAKES 4 SERVINGS
(¾ cup each)

....

1 cup (193 g) uncooked teff
¼ teaspoon cloves
¼ teaspoon allspice
3 cups (711 ml) boiling water
⅓ cup (49 g) chopped dates
⅓ cup (50 g) chopped dried figs
⅓ cup (41 g) pistachios
Plant-based milk, optional

1. Heat a heavy pot over medium heat. Add the teff, cloves, and allspice and toast, stirring constantly, for 5 minutes, until the teff pops and smells fragrant.

2. Carefully remove the pot from the heat and add the boiling water slowly to avoid splattering. Stir in the water and place the pot back on the burner. Cook over medium heat for about 15 minutes, stirring with a whisk occasionally to avoid lumping and sticking.

3. Remove the pan from the heat and stir in the dates, figs, and pistachios. Serve with plant-based milk, if desired.

note: You can make a big batch of this porridge and reheat it for breakfast the next morning in the microwave. If you plan on doing this, add the dates, figs, and pistachios right before serving the cereal to avoid sogginess.

variations: Substitute chopped fresh figs for the dried figs, or almonds or walnuts for the pistachios.

PER SERVING: 310 calories, 9 g protein, 58 g carbohydrate, 6 g fat, 1 g saturated fat, 6 g fiber, 10 g sugar, 77 mg sodium
STAR NUTRIENTS: thiamin (13% DV), vitamin B6 (12% DV), calcium (14% DV), copper (21% DV), iron (26% DV), magnesium (24% DV), manganese (250% DV), phosphorus (22% DV), potassium (10% DV), zinc (12% DV)

Harvest Wild Rice Salad with
Persimmons and Baby Spinach

Eat a dark green leafy vegetable every day.

Harvest Wild Rice Salad with Persimmons and Baby Spinach
Tuscan Fusilli with Swiss Chard and Fava Beans

Long before dark green leaves were available prewashed and precut in convenient bags in the supermarket produce aisle, people foraged in forests, jungles, and meadows for wild greens in order to lend a pungent, flavorful bite and potent nutrients to their diets—a practice that continues to this day. Nearly every culture has food traditions surrounding wild greens: wild nettles in Turkey and amaranth leaves in parts of India. Recently, Westerners have participated in a resurgence of discovering wild greens in their own neighborhood woods, such as dandelion, mustard, watercress, sorrel, purslane, and poke.

But you don't have to root around outdoors for wild greens if you don't want to; an increasing variety of greens are available in supermarkets, farmers markets, and CSAs, including mustard greens, collard greens, kale, spinach, bok choy, turnip greens, beet greens, watercress, romaine lettuce, green leaf lettuce, and arugula. The nutrition profile of dark green leafy vegetables is off the charts; that's why I recommend you include a serving in your diet every day. These plants are rich in essential vitamins and minerals, including calcium—which can be a challenge for the plant-powered eater to obtain—and phytochemicals, such as beta-carotene, lutein, zeaxanthin, and chlorophyll. No wonder green leafy vegetables have been linked with reducing inflammation and oxidation, thus promoting heart and bone health and even helping to protect against age-related eye disease and cognitive decline.

Make sure each day includes a healthy dose (½ cup cooked or 1 cup raw) of green leafy vegetables. Sauté greens as a side dish or a topping for tortillas, grits, or grains; toss tender baby greens into salads; and stir greens into soups, stews, and casseroles.

See photo
on page 168

harvest wild rice salad with persimmons and baby spinach

ACTIVE PREPARATION TIME: 20 minutes • **TOTAL PREPARATION TIME: 45 minutes**

Harness the power of greens every day—even when the cool weather descends. This harvest salad calls upon deep-green spinach, gorgeous fall persimmons, and a tahini-ginger dressing for a hearty flavor (and nutrition) punch. Packed with slow-burning carbs, heart-loving fats and antioxidants, and powerful plant protein, you can tuck this salad away in a container for a satisfying lunch on the go, or serve it for dinner with chili or a simple bean dish, such as Rosemary and Olive Cassoulet (page 86). This salad is proof that you don't have to skimp on flavor and pizzazz when summer's produce bounty is at its end!

MAKES 8 SERVINGS
(about 1⅛ cups each)

½ cup (93 g) uncooked brown basmati rice
½ cup (80 g) uncooked wild rice
2¼ cups (533 ml) water
3 medium firm persimmons, coarsely chopped
1 cup (101 g) diced celery
½ cup (30 g) chopped fresh parsley
2 green onions, white and green parts, sliced
½ cup (58 g) coarsely chopped walnuts
¼ cup (41 g) dried cranberries
2 tablespoons tahini (see Note)
4 tablespoons lemon juice
1 teaspoon honey or agave nectar
½ teaspoon stone-ground mustard
1 teaspoon caraway seeds
½ teaspoon minced fresh ginger
¼ teaspoon black pepper
Pinch of sea salt, optional
1½ cups (47 g) baby spinach leaves

1. Combine the brown basmati rice and wild rice in a small pot. Add the water, cover, and bring to a boil. Reduce to medium heat and cook for 40 minutes, until tender. Allow to cool slightly.

2. While the rice is cooking, combine the persimmons, celery, parsley, green onions, walnuts, and cranberries in a medium bowl.

3. In a small dish, whisk together the tahini, lemon juice, honey, mustard, caraway seeds, ginger, and black pepper. Taste and add a pinch of sea salt, if desired.

4. Add the cooled rice to the persimmon mixture. Add the dressing to the salad and toss.

5. Line a salad bowl or platter with the spinach. Spoon the rice salad over it and serve immediately.

note: Tahini, sometimes called sesame seed paste, is available at most natural food and Mediterranean markets, as well as many large grocery stores.

variations: Substitute another whole grain, such as quinoa, barley, bulgur, or farro for the brown rice, following package directions for cooking instructions. If you can't find persimmons, substitute sliced fresh or canned (drained) peaches. Omit the spinach to create a grain-based salad that will store for up to 3 days in the refrigerator.

> **PER SERVING:** 172 calories, 5 g protein, 24 g carbohydrate, 7 g fat, 1 g saturated fat, 3 g fiber, 2 g sugar, 30 mg sodium
> **STAR NUTRIENTS:** folate (12% DV), thiamin (10% DV), vitamin A (23% DV), vitamin C (27% DV), vitamin K (129% DV), copper (18% DV), iron (11% DV), magnesium (14% DV), phosphorus (14% DV), selenium (10% DV)

tuscan fusilli with swiss chard and fava beans

ACTIVE PREPARATION TIME: **13 minutes** • TOTAL PREPARATION TIME: **20 minutes**

Green leafy vegetables are brimming with good health and flavor, and are also a classic ingredient in many traditional dishes, such as this simple Tuscan pasta. Since most of the other ingredients—whole grain fusilli, sun-dried tomatoes, canned beans, onion, garlic, and spices—can be kept on hand, you can whip up this rustic one-dish meal in minutes. Just pick up some Swiss chard and mushrooms at the farmers market or supermarket, and you're good to go. That's why this budget-friendly meal should become one of your favorite go-to meals on those busy nights—you'll get in your daily greens allotment faster than you could order takeout!

MAKES 8 SERVINGS
(about 1⅛ cups each)

4 cups (948 ml) water
8 ounces (227 g) uncooked whole grain fusilli pasta
1 tablespoon extra virgin olive oil
½ medium onion, diced
3 medium garlic cloves, minced
1½ teaspoons dried oregano
¼ teaspoon smoked paprika (see Notes)
1½ cups (105 g) sliced mushrooms
¼ cup (14 g) sun-dried tomatoes, chopped
One 15-ounce (425 g) can fava beans, no salt added, rinsed and drained (see Notes)
One 10-ounce (284 g) bunch rainbow Swiss chard, sliced (about 9 loosely packed cups; see Notes)
Pinch of kosher salt, optional

1. Fill a medium pot with the water, cover, and bring to a boil over high heat. Decrease the heat to medium, add the pasta, and cook for 7 minutes, until al dente. Drain the pasta and return to the pot, covered, to keep warm.
2. While the pasta is cooking, heat the olive oil in a large skillet or sauté pan over medium heat. Add the onions, garlic, oregano, and paprika and sauté for 4 minutes.
3. Add the mushrooms, tomatoes, and fava beans and sauté for an additional 3 minutes.
4. Add the Swiss chard and cover the pan. Cook for 2 minutes, then remove the lid and cook, stirring, for an additional 2 minutes—just until the chard is wilted but still bright green.

5. Stir the pasta into the vegetables in the pan to heat through. Taste and add a pinch of kosher salt, if desired.
6. Serve immediately.

notes: Decrease or increase the amount of paprika to adjust the dish's zest. If you'd like to use fava beans cooked from scratch, add 1¾ cups in step 3.

If rainbow chard is not available, try another variety, such as traditional green Swiss chard, or substitute another green, such as dandelion or mustard greens. If you'd like to use frozen greens, add 10 ounces, thawed and drained, in step 4 and cook just until heated through.

variations: You may substitute any other pasta shape, such as fettuccine, rotini, or farfalle (cook according to package directions). You may also replace the fava beans with another kind, such as cannellini, kidney, or an heirloom variety.

PER SERVING: 178 calories, 9 g protein, 33 g carbohydrate, 3 g fat, .5 g saturated fat, 6 g fiber, 4 g sugar, 105 mg sodium
STAR NUTRIENTS: folate (15% DV), niacin (15% DV), riboflavin (15% DV), thiamin (17% DV), vitamin A (47% DV), vitamin C (39% DV), vitamin K (144% DV), copper (17% DV), iron (16% DV), magnesium (24% DV), manganese (27% DV), potassium (12% DV)

Moroccan Vegetable
Tagine with Couscous

Spice it up!

Muhammara
Red Lentil Soup with Root Vegetables and Sage
Moroccan Vegetable Tagine with Couscous

In India, a home cook might sprinkle more than a dozen different herbs and spices, such as turmeric, fenugreek and cumin, into her cooking pots for dinner. And in Thailand, a dish may call upon a long list of aromatic herbs and spices, such as lemongrass, basil, and chilies. Throughout history, spices have been regarded as precious; they were collected, traded, and even used as currency. They literally "launched a thousand ships" (or more) in the spice trade between Asia, Africa, and Europe that dates back to antiquity. Today, they are still beloved around the world.

Pinches of spices (the buds, bark, roots, berries, seeds, or stigmas of plants) and snippets of herbs (the leaves of plants) provide so much vibrant, bold taste to foods. Imagine how overjoyed our early ancestors must have been when they discovered the flavor that a handful of wild garlic or cilantro could bring to a bland stew bubbling on the fire. Serendipitously, herbs and spices also offer more than great taste: they are concentrated sources of antioxidant and anti-inflammatory compounds. These plant foods have been used as natural medicine for millennia, and modern science agrees: their benefits seem to include antimicrobial action, cancer-fighting properties, and even brain protection.

Don't be shy of herbs and spices—using them is one of the most significant and economical culinary choices you can ever make! For just a few dollars, bottles of thyme, paprika, and cinnamon can offer potent flavor and nutrition to hundreds of meals. Start sprinkling a variety of spices and handfuls of fresh herbs into soups, stews, salads, entrées, side dishes, and even desserts. Spice blends, such as low-sodium herbal blends (commercially available in most supermarkets) and special blends, such as herbes de Provence and Cajun seasoning blends may be purchased premixed, or you can make your own (see page 345). These blends are already designed to suit traditional dishes from those cuisines.

There are no set rules for pairing spices with plant foods, although you may want to avoid mixing too many strong spices and herbs together in one dish. Let the pages of this book serve as an inspiration for learning how to glorify the flavors of plant foods with aromatic herbs and spices, as nearly every recipe calls upon these potent plant flavorings. If you have the space and want to give it a try, grow some herbs in a pot on your doorstep or windowsill. They may not be the magical ingredients our ancestors imagined, but these bold plant foods are sure to enchant you.

muhammara

ACTIVE PREPARATION TIME: **9 minutes** • TOTAL PREPARATION TIME: **9 minutes**

Fill your foods with the essence of spice. It's easy. Just take this classic dip, which originates from Syria and is traditionally served in Palestinian and Lebanese cuisine. The rich color and flavors come from roasted red peppers, walnuts, spices, and pomegranate molasses—a pomegranate juice concentrate featured in many Middle Eastern dishes. Serve it with whole wheat pita and vegetables as a dip, or as a spread in sandwiches and wraps.

MAKES 10 SERVINGS
(about ¼ cup each)

One 12-ounce (340 g) jar roasted red peppers, drained (2 tablespoons liquid reserved)
2 tablespoons tomato paste
1 tablespoon lemon juice
1½ tablespoons extra virgin olive oil
2 tablespoons pomegranate molasses (see Notes)
1 cup (116 g) chopped toasted walnuts
½ cup (34 g) whole grain bread crumbs (see Note on page 95)
1 teaspoon crushed red pepper, or more to taste
1 teaspoon cumin
½ teaspoon allspice
2 tablespoons chopped fresh parsley

1. Place the roasted red peppers, reserved liquid, tomato paste, lemon juice, olive oil, pomegranate molasses, walnuts, bread crumbs, crushed red pepper, cumin, and allspice in a blender. Process until smooth, scraping down the sides as needed.
2. Pour the blender contents into a serving dish and sprinkle with the parsley.
3. Serve with pita chips, fresh vegetables, or bread as a spread or dip.

notes: Look for pomegranate molasses—essentially boiled-down pomegranate juice—in specialty food stores, Middle Eastern markets, or online. If you can't find it, substitute half honey and half balsamic vinegar (although the flavor will be different).

Store leftovers in an airtight container in the fridge for up to 1 week.

PER SERVING: 129 calories, 3 g protein, 9 g carbohydrate, 10 g fat, 1 g saturated fat, 2 g fiber, 3 g sugar, 83 mg sodium
STAR NUTRIENTS: vitamin A (23% DV), vitamin C (30% DV), vitamin K (17% DV), copper (10% DV), manganese (26% DV)

red lentil soup with root vegetables and sage

ACTIVE PREPARATION TIME: **15 minutes** • TOTAL PREPARATION TIME: **1 hour**

This savory soup, rich in carotenoid antioxidants, is a bright, sunny shade of orange—the perfect way to cheer up the cloudiest of days. Its herbal flavor—which includes the warm flavors of the Mediterranean spices sage and smoked paprika—and hearty texture make it ideal to pair with a salad, such as Haricots Verts, Tomato, and Almond Salad (page 32) or a sandwich half. When it comes to crafting delicious soups, it's all about letting spices and herbs infuse each bowl with tantalizing taste and aroma, as well as potent antioxidant and anti-inflammatory properties that can boost disease protection.

MAKES 8 SERVINGS
(about 1 cup each)

6 cups (1,422 ml) water
One 14.5-ounce (411 g) can diced tomatoes, no salt added, with liquid
1 teaspoon reduced sodium vegetable broth base
1 small onion, diced
½ medium bell pepper (red, yellow, or orange), diced
1 cup celery, chopped
2 medium carrots, chopped
2 small red potatoes, diced
2 medium garlic cloves, minced
1 cup (192 g) dried red lentils
1½ teaspoons dried sage
½ teaspoon low-sodium herbal seasoning blend (see page 345)
½ teaspoon smoked paprika

1. Combine the water and tomatoes in a large pot on the stovetop. Stir in the broth base and turn the heat to medium-high.

2. Add the onion, bell pepper, celery, carrots, potatoes, garlic, red lentils, sage, herbal seasoning, and paprika.

3. Stir well, cover, and bring to a boil. Reduce the heat to medium and simmer for 40 to 45 minutes, until the vegetables are tender. Add water as needed to replace moisture lost to evaporation, although the consistency should be thick and hearty.

note: To prepare in a slow cooker, combine all ingredients and cook 4 to 5 hours on high or 8 to 10 hours on low.

variations: Substitute another variety of lentil, such as beluga or green, for the red lentils.

PER SERVING: 141 calories, 8 g protein, 27 g carbohydrate, 0 g fat, 0 g saturated fat, 10 g fiber, 4 g sugar, 25 mg sodium

STAR NUTRIENTS: folate (34% DV), thiamin (17% DV), vitamin A (49% DV), vitamin B6 (14% DV), vitamin C (53% DV), vitamin K (17% DV), iron (13% DV), magnesium (11% DV), potassium (15% DV)

---

moroccan vegetable tagine
with couscous

Revel in the exotic tastes and smells of spices, which can boost your diet with anti-inflammatory power. North African in origin, a tagine is a flavorful, vegetable-infused stew named after the clay pot in which it is traditionally cooked and served. This version highlights sweet potatoes, tomatoes, eggplant, and cauliflower—liberally seasoned with Moroccan spices, including cumin, turmeric, and cardamom. Serve it with Edamame Hummus (page 148) and whole wheat pita bread.

MAKES 8 SERVINGS
(about 1⅓ cups each)

....

Tagine
1 tablespoon extra virgin olive oil
1 medium onion, chopped
2 medium garlic cloves, minced
1 teaspoon minced fresh ginger
3 tablespoons harissa (see Notes)
2 teaspoons cumin
½ teaspoon cardamom
1 teaspoon coriander
½ teaspoon turmeric
¼ teaspoon black pepper
2 tablespoons tomato paste
1½ cups (355 ml) reduced sodium vegetable broth (see Notes
    on page 346)
One 14.5-ounce (411 g) can diced tomatoes, no salt added, with
    liquid
One 15-ounce (425 g) can chickpeas, no salt added, rinsed and
    drained (or 1¾ cups cooked)
2 medium sweet potatoes, chopped
2 medium carrots, sliced
½ small head cauliflower, chopped into small florets (about 1⅓
    cups or 133 g)
½ medium eggplant, diced into small cubes

Couscous and Toppings
2 cups (474 ml) water
2 cups (346 g) uncooked whole grain couscous
¼ cup (41 g) raisins, not packed
¼ cup (33 g) chopped dried apricots, not packed

1. Lower the baking rack in the oven to accommodate the tagine (see Notes) and preheat the oven to 350°F (180°C).

2. In a large, ovenproof tagine with a lid (11 inches across), combine the olive oil, onion, garlic, ginger, harissa, cumin, cardamom, coriander, turmeric, black pepper, tomato paste, broth, tomatoes, chickpeas, sweet potatoes, carrots, cauliflower and eggplant. Stir well. Cover and bake for 1½ hours, stirring every 30 minutes, until vegetables are tender.

3. About 10 minutes before serving, bring the water to a boil in a medium pot. When boiling, remove from the heat and add the couscous. Cover the pot and set aside for 5 minutes, then lift the lid, toss the couscous with a fork, and transfer it to a serving dish.

4. Remove the lid from the tagine and sprinkle with the raisins and apricots. Serve the tagine over the couscous.

notes: Harissa is a traditional North African condiment made of chiles that provides an essential flavor to this dish. You can usually find it in Mediterranean markets, as well as some gourmet food stores, international markets, and online purveyors.

You can find a tagine in many kitchen stores, but if you don't have one, use a deep casserole dish or Dutch oven with a tight-fitting lid.

variations: Substitute 1⅓ cups cooked lentils or beans for the chickpeas, or add 8 ounces (227 g) diced firm tofu (pressed, for best results—see page 103), if desired. To make this gluten-free, use brown rice couscous.

PER SERVING: 340 calories, 13 g protein, 67 g carbohydrate, 5 g fat, .5 g saturated fat, 13 g fiber, 15 g sugar, 230 mg sodium
STAR NUTRIENTS: folate (14% DV), vitamin A (142% DV), vitamin B6 (10% DV), vitamin C (68% DV), iron (18% DV), magnesium (11% DV), manganese (16% DV), potassium (18% DV)

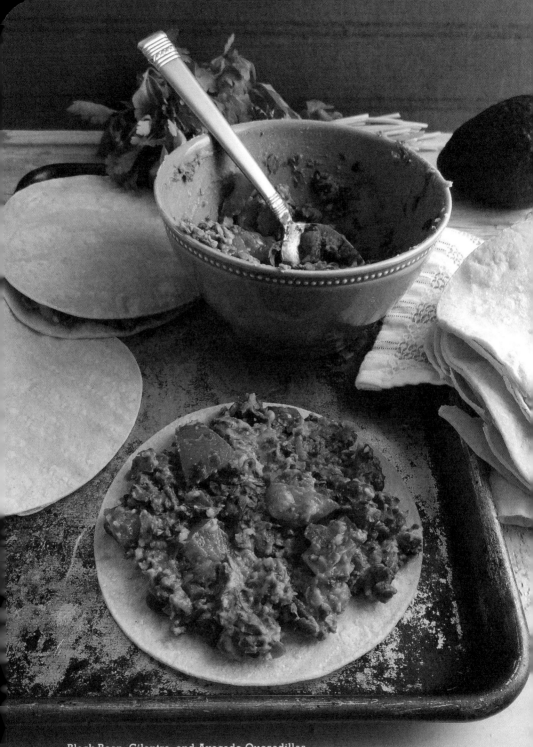

Black Bean, Cilantro, and Avocado Quesadillas

Ditch the salt, power up on real flavor.

Black Bean, Cilantro, and Avocado Quesadillas
Rustic White Bean and Sun-Dried Tomato Toasts

❦

Trans fats, pesticides, added sugar—these are the things that get lots of attention when you shop for food. But what about salt? Most of the time, it takes the back seat when you scan nutrition labels. However, it's one of the most important health issues many of us face.

We are eating way too much sodium (the main constituent of salt): on average 3,400 milligrams a day, though we should be limiting it to less than 2,300 milligrams, or 1 teaspoon of salt, a day. What's wrong with eating so much salt? It can put you at risk for high blood pressure, which in turn raises your risk for heart disease and stroke.

Most of that sodium in your diet isn't coming from real food, like carrots, celery, oats, and beans. Our high sodium intake isn't even primarily due to the saltshaker; instead, processed and prepared foods make up a whopping 77 percent of our daily sodium intake. One of the most beneficial things you can do for your health is to start cooking whole plant foods—naturally low in sodium—and season them with a collection of herbs and spices for natural pizzazz minus the sodium (see page 345). Skip the packaged, prepared foods—food manufacturers will almost always add more sodium than you would—and make it yourself.

I don't list salt as a required ingredient in my recipes, because I want you to discover the real flavor of foods, without the addition of salt to mask them. During my culinary training, I learned a trick from chefs: they rarely measure out salt for a recipe. Instead, they usually keep a saltcellar (small pot of good quality sea or kosher salt) on the countertop, and as they taste a dish, they add a pinch (or two or three).

Start applying this lesson to your own cooking, using my recipes as a guide. Many are so potent in flavor, you'll find no salt called for. Other recipes benefit from just a pinch of salt—about one-eighth of a teaspoon (288 milligrams of sodium) for the whole dish. So, take the cookbook phrase "to taste" literally and taste every dish before you add any salt; let the real flavors of plant foods shine on their own.

See photo
on page 182

black bean, cilantro, and avocado quesadillas

I think fresh Mexican foods make up some of the most delicious plant-powered meals in the universe. Take these easy quesadillas—a simple solution for getting a healthy meal on the table in 30 minutes that the entire family will enjoy. And who needs added salt when the flavors of cilantro, garlic, chile, and lemon juice shine through?

MAKES 4 SERVINGS
(1 quesadilla each)

One 15-ounce (425 g) can black beans, no salt added, rinsed and drained, liquid reserved (or 1¾ cups cooked)
1 medium tomato, diced
½ small chile pepper (e.g., jalapeño, Anaheim), finely diced
1 tablespoon fresh lemon juice
1 medium garlic clove, minced
¼ cup (15 g) finely diced fresh cilantro
2 teaspoons extra virgin olive oil
Eight 6-inch (15 cm) corn tortillas
¼ cup (28 g) plant-based shredded cheese, optional
1 medium avocado, peeled and cut into thin slices
Plant-based sour cream, optional (see page 344)

1. In a small mixing bowl, mash the beans with a potato masher or fork, adding 1 to 2 tablespoons of the reserved bean liquid to make a thick, lumpy mixture.
2. Add the tomato, chile pepper, lemon juice, garlic, and cilantro to the beans and mix well.
3. Heat 1 teaspoon of the olive oil in a large skillet.
4. Spread ½ cup of the bean mixture onto 2 tortillas smoothly. Place them in the skillet, bean side up. Sprinkle each with 1 tablespoon of plant-based cheese, if desired. Top with another tortilla. Cook the quesadillas over medium heat for about 4 minutes, until the bottom side is browned. Turn over carefully and cook the other side for about 4 minutes, until browned.
5. Remove the quesadilla from the skillet and garnish with avocado slices and plant-based sour cream, if desired. Repeat the process again to make 4 quesadillas.

variation: You may substitute canned pinto beans or white beans for the black beans, or use 1¾ cups cooked beans or lentils (any variety). If you don't like cilantro, you may substitute parsley.

PER SERVING: 302 calories, 9 g protein, 47 g carbohydrate, 12 g fat, 2 g saturated fat, 12 g fiber, 4 g sugar, 282 mg sodium
STAR NUTRIENTS: folate (26% DV), vitamin B6 (15% DV), vitamin C (36% DV), calcium (18% DV), iron (16% DV), magnesium (13% DV), phosphorus (23% DV), potassium (22% DV)

rustic white bean and sun-dried tomato toasts

ACTIVE PREPARATION TIME: **15 minutes** • TOTAL PREPARATION TIME: **20 minutes**

These zesty toasts, spread with bean dip and sun-dried tomatoes, are a simple appetizer for a gathering, or an accompaniment for a large crock of vegetable soup, such as Borscht with Beets and Beet Greens (page 000). You won't even miss the salt when your tongue is greeted by the intense flavors of garlic, black pepper, lemon juice, and basil.

MAKES 8 SERVINGS
(1 toast each)

....

One 15-ounce (425 g) can cannellini beans, no salt added,
   rinsed and drained (or 1¾ cups cooked)
½ tablespoon extra virgin olive oil
2 medium garlic cloves, minced
¼ teaspoon freshly ground black pepper
1½ tablespoons fresh lemon juice
Eight 1-ounce (28 g) slices rustic whole grain bread
8 fresh basil leaves
½ cup (28 g) chopped sun-dried tomatoes

1. Preheat the oven to 400°F (205°C).

2. In a medium bowl, mix together the beans, olive oil, garlic, black pepper, and lemon juice. Mash the bean mixture with a potato masher or fork until thick and lumpy.

3. Arrange the bread slices on a baking sheet. Bake for about 5 minutes, until toasted and lightly golden. Remove from the oven.

4. Prepare each toast by spreading 2½ tablespoons of bean spread onto each slice and topping it with a basil leaf and 1 tablespoon of the sun-dried tomatoes.

note: Prepare this bean dip in step 2, without the additional ingredients or steps, as a tasty accompaniment to whole grain pita or fresh vegetables.

variation: Substitute 1¾ cups cooked chickpeas, lentils, or beans for the cannellini beans.

PER SERVING: 149 calories, 7 g protein, 27 g carbohydrate, 1.5 g fat, 0 g saturated fat, 4 g fiber, 3 sugar, 161 mg sodium

STAR NUTRIENTS: folate (14% DV), niacin (20% DV), thiamin (11% DV), vitamin C (12% DV), vitamin K (11% DV), copper (21% DV), iron (11% DV), magnesium (16% DV), manganese (66% DV), potassium (10% DV), selenium (15% DV)

Chana Dal Stew

Eat your way to the end of the rainbow.

Blueberry Oatmeal Waffles
Apple and Fennel Salad with Arugula
Chana Dal Stew
🦃

Plants come in an astonishing array of vibrant colors, from sunny yellow and spring green to bright scarlet and deep purple-black. In many cases, these colors helped ensure the survival of the plant. Our ancestors could spot them against a canopy of leaves, making it a cinch to pluck the fruits, eat them, and spit out their seeds along their journey, ensuring the next generation of plant life.

Natural pigments, from anthocyanin's purple-blue-black hue to lycopene's scarlet shade, color the flesh and skins of plants. And these natural colorants in the plant are categorized as phytochemicals, bioactive plant compounds that possess health benefits. In the past few decades, scientists have isolated thousands of phytochemicals, and they are adding to their discoveries about these compounds every day.

Plants could not get up and run away from their predators or environmental threats, such as insects and the sun. Instead, they evolved a powerful defense system in their skin and flesh to protect themselves from insects, viruses, and UV damage—a complex array of phytochemicals. Now we know that these phytochemicals, which have anti-inflammatory and antioxidant action, offer us protection when we eat them in plants. The lycopene found in tomatoes may protect against prostate cancer, and lutein in corn may help prevent age-related eye disease. There's a similar story to tell for dozens of phytochemicals.

The moral: mow through colorful plants every day, including white (e.g., potatoes, mushrooms, turnips), yellow (e.g., corn, summer squash, lemons), orange (e.g., squash, carrots, oranges), red (e.g., tomatoes, watermelon, red peppers), blue-purple (e.g., blueberries, eggplant, black beans), and green (e.g., spinach, zucchini, broccoli).

blueberry oatmeal waffles

ACTIVE PREPARATION TIME: **14 minutes** • TOTAL PREPARATION TIME: **40 minutes**

The deep purple-blue of blueberries is a calling card for their rich phyto-chemical stash. Blueberries are rich in a number of these health-protective plant compounds, in particular anthocyanins, which have been linked to all sorts of benefits—even brain health. When fresh blueberries aren't in season, use frozen or dried, as in this scrumptious waffle recipe.

MAKES 6 SERVINGS
(1 large waffle each)

1½ cups (356 ml) unsweetened plain plant-based milk
2 tablespoons chia seeds (see Notes on page 139)
3 tablespoons canola oil, expeller pressed
1 tablespoon maple syrup
½ cups (60 g) unsweetened dried blueberries
1¼ cups (150 g) white whole wheat flour
½ cup (78 g) uncooked old-fashioned oats
1 tablespoon baking powder
1 teaspoon cinnamon
⅓ cup (39 g) chopped walnuts
Nonstick cooking spray

1. In a medium bowl, using a wire whisk or electric mixer, mix together the plant-based milk, chia seeds, canola oil, and maple syrup for 2 minutes. Mix in the dried blueberries.

2. In a separate bowl, toss together the flour, oats, baking powder, cinnamon, and walnuts until mixed well. Add the flour mixture to the milk mixture and stir just until combined; do not overmix.

3. Heat a 7-inch waffle iron on the medium-low setting.

4. Spray the waffle iron with nonstick cooking spray. Place ½ cup of batter onto the waffle iron and spread it over the surface. Cook the waffle for about 7 minutes, until cooked through and golden brown. Repeat, spraying iron with cooking spray between each waffle, until all waffles are cooked.

variations: Substitute dried cranberries, cherries, or strawberries for the blueberries. To make this gluten-free, substitute 1 cup of an all-purpose gluten-free flour blend (e.g., Bob's Red Mill or King Arthur Flour) for the 1¼ cups white whole wheat flour and check that all other ingredients are gluten-free.

PER SERVING: 295 calories, 8 g protein, 38 g carbohydrate, 14 g fat, 1 g saturated fat, 6 g fiber, 11 g sugar, 27 mg sodium
STAR NUTRIENTS: riboflavin (13% DV), thiamin (17% DV), calcium (23% DV), copper (14% DV), iron (12% DV), magnesium (17% DV), manganese (77% DV), phosphorus (34% DV), potassium (13% DV), selenium (46% DV)

apple and fennel salad with arugula

ACTIVE PREPARATION TIME: **10 minutes** • TOTAL PREPARATION TIME: **10 minutes**

Licoricelike fennel adds a crisp bite to this cool-weather salad of apples, walnuts, arugula, and a Dijon-apple vinaigrette. Packed with color—deep green leaves, rose-colored fruit, and pale white-green bulbs—this salad is also rich in many phytochemicals, offering a welcome boost for your health—and spirits—on the dreariest day. Pair it with a comfort-food dish, such as Smoky Chili with Sweet Potatoes (page 198). It's also delicious packed up for lunch the next day.

MAKES 6 SERVINGS
(about 1¼ cups each)

- 4 cups (80 g) packed arugula leaves, washed, drained
- 1 medium crisp red or pink apple (such as Fuji or Honeycrisp), unpeeled, thinly sliced
- 1 medium fennel bulb, trimmed, halved, and thinly sliced
- 1 tablespoon extra virgin olive oil
- 2 tablespoons apple juice
- ½ tablespoon apple cider vinegar
- ¼ teaspoon freshly ground black pepper
- ½ teaspoon low-sodium herbal seasoning blend (see page 345)
- 1 teaspoon Dijon mustard
- ⅓ cup (39 g) chopped walnuts

1. Place the arugula in a large bowl. Add the apples and fennel.
2. Whisk together the olive oil, apple juice, vinegar, black pepper, herbal seasoning, and mustard in a small dish. Drizzle over the salad and toss well.
3. Sprinkle with the chopped walnuts. Serve immediately.

variations: You may substitute baby spinach for the arugula; pear for the apple; and pecans, hazelnuts, or almonds for the walnuts.

PER SERVING: 96 calories, 2 g protein, 9 g carbohydrate, 7 g fat, 1 g saturated fat, 3 g fiber, 4 g sugar, 45 mg sodium
STAR NUTRIENTS: vitamin C (13% DV), vitamin K (35% DV)

---

chana dal stew

See photo
on page 188

ACTIVE PREPARATION TIME: **12 minutes** • TOTAL PREPARATION TIME: **1 hour**

This spicy, flavorful stew's structure is based on chana dal—split, polished baby chickpeas. Dal, which means "split grain," is a classic Indian dish featuring simmered legumes, such as lentils. The golden spices and orange-red root vegetables, packed with plant carotenoids linked with heart health, further accentuate this amber legume. Best of all, just toss all of the ingredients into a pot and it will be done in less than an hour. Serve it with a cool grain salad, such as Bombay Carrot, Beet, and Bulgur Salad (page 142).

MAKES 6 SERVINGS
(about 1 cup each)

8 ounces (227 g or 1¼ cups) dried chana dal
5 cups (711 ml) water
2 medium carrots, sliced
1 medium red bell pepper, chopped
1 medium onion, chopped
2 small red potatoes, unpeeled, chopped
2 small tomatoes, chopped
1 teaspoon garam masala (see page 345)
½ teaspoon turmeric
½ teaspoon grated fresh ginger
2 medium garlic cloves, minced
¼ teaspoon crushed red pepper
1 tablespoon unsalted creamy peanut butter

1. Place all ingredients in a large pot, stir well, cover, and bring to a simmer.
2. Cook for about 50 minutes, until the vegetables and chana dal are tender.

note: You may also cook this dish in a slow cooker on high for 4 to 5 hours or on low for 8 to 10 hours.

variation: Substitute red or yellow lentils for the chana dal and reduce the cooking time by about 15 minutes.

PER SERVING: 215 calories, 12 g protein, 40 g carbohydrate, 1 g fat, 0 g saturated fat, 14 g fiber, 4 g sugar, 34 mg sodium
STAR NUTRIENTS: folate (53% DV), niacin (13% DV), thiamin (28% DV), vitamin A (94% DV), vitamin B6 (22% DV), vitamin C (51% DV), iron (24% DV), magnesium (20% DV), potassium (26% DV), zinc (15% DV)

Smoky Chili with
Sweet Potatoes

Invest in the money- and time-saving kitchen tools you need.

Smoky Chili with Sweet Potatoes
Pigeon Peas with Pumpkin and Sofrito

One of the fears that people face when they consider adopting a healthy plant-powered eating style is the extra time required in the kitchen. After all, vegetables need to be chopped, beans need to be soaked, and whole grains need to be cooked. It's hard to cook up dried beans or whole grains for a quick dinner on the spur of the moment, and it always takes longer than you expected to chop up fresh vegetables for a stir-fry.

Today's supermarkets offer many time-saving products for the plant-based kitchen, including prechopped vegetables and fruits and precooked pouches of grains and legumes. But these products come at a premium. Still, considering that animal protein is one of the most expensive items in the supermarket, a plant-powered diet can be very economical, especially if you fill your shopping cart with simple staples like dried beans, oats, seasonal produce, and nuts.

To use those economical staples, you should enlist some powerful kitchen tools as your ally. Remember, you don't have to buy top-of-the-line kitchen utensils; simple versions may be found at a reasonable cost. In addition to the basics—sharp knives in a few sizes, wire whisks, mixing spoons, spatulas, measuring spoons and cups, and cutting boards—here are a few of my favorite kitchen tools:

- **Slow cooker.** Though this handy device is often associated with cooking meat, it's also perfect for the plant-powered kitchen: just toss in soaked beans, whole grains, vegetables, broth, herbs, and spices, push the button, and when you get home a one-dish meal is waiting for you. A 3-quart cooker is the perfect size to accommodate the plant-powered recipes in this book. As a general rule of thumb, if a recipe takes 1 to 2 hours to make in the oven or stovetop, it will take 4 to 6 hours on the high setting or 8 to 10 hours on low.
- **Pressure cooker.** Today's pressure cookers are sleek, safe, and easy—and, best of all, fast! You can cook soaked beans in about 10

minutes instead of an hour or more on the stove, unsoaked beans in about 25 minutes instead of soaking overnight before cooking, and whole grains in about 20 minutes instead of about an hour on the stove. See page 23 and page 65 for more on legumes and grains.

◄ **Food processor, chopper, blender, or immersion blender.** Though you *can* get by without these devices, I suggest buying at least one of them. Even the budget-friendliest varieties can help you chop large amounts of vegetables for soups or stir-fries, grind nuts into nut butters, puree herbs into pesto, turn dairy-free soups creamy, and whip up a fruity smoothie in seconds. Your first purchase might be a blender (or immersion blender) to liquefy or combine ingredients, followed by a small food chopper to help chop up vegetables.

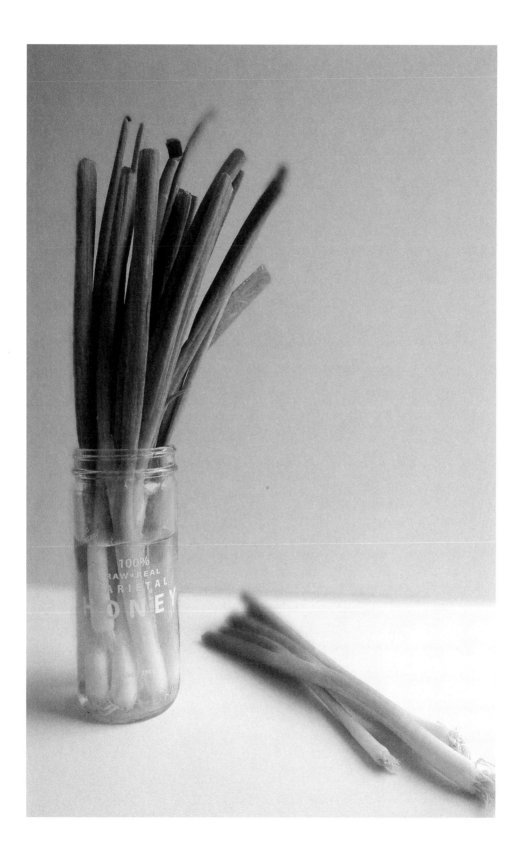

See photo
on page 194

smoky chili with sweet potatoes

ACTIVE PREPARATION TIME: **16 minutes** • TOTAL PREPARATION TIME: **1 hour 5 minutes**
(not including soaking time)

Looking for an easy way to put economical, plant-powered meals on the table? No sweat! Just invest in a slow cooker to simmer a number of dishes—all you've got to do is throw in the ingredients, set the dial, and walk away. The smoky, golden notes—rich in heart-healthy beta-carotene—in this chili make it a fall favorite perfect for a potluck or tailgate party. Pair it with Seeded Whole Wheat Biscuits (page 210) and a salad for a simple meal. The leftovers are great the next day, too!

MAKES 10 SERVINGS
(about 1 cup each)

2 cups (368 g) dried small red beans (e.g., anasazi or kidney)
4½ cups (1,067 ml) water, plus more for soaking
1 teaspoon reduced sodium vegetable broth base
One 14.5-ounce (411 g) can fire-roasted diced tomatoes, no salt
    added, with liquid
2 tablespoons tomato paste
1 medium yellow onion, diced
2 medium sweet potatoes, diced
3 celery stalks, diced
2 medium garlic cloves, minced
1 teaspoon smoked paprika
1 teaspoon chili powder
1 teaspoon cumin
1 teaspoon liquid smoke (see Notes)

1. Cover the beans with water and soak overnight.

2. Drain the beans and add to a large pot with the 4½ cups of water and the broth base. Bring to a boil, covered, over medium-high heat, then reduce the heat to medium and simmer for 20 minutes.

3. Add the tomatoes, tomato paste, onion, sweet potatoes, celery, garlic, paprika, chili powder, cumin, and liquid smoke and stir well. Cover and cook for an additional 40 to 45 minutes, stirring occasionally, until the sweet potatoes are tender yet firm and the beans are tender. Add water as needed to replace moisture lost to evaporation, although the consistency should be thick.

notes: Liquid smoke is available in many supermarkets in the spice or seasoning section; it is made by smoking wood and collecting the condensed droplets, so it adds a wonderful smokiness to dishes.

To prepare the dish in a slow cooker, place the soaked beans and the remaining ingredients into the container and cook for 4 to 5 hours on high or 8 to 10 hours on low.

variation: Substitute dried white beans, garbanzo beans, or heirloom beans for the red beans.

PER SERVING: 167 calories, 10 g protein, 32 g carbohydrate, .5 g fat, 0 g saturated fat, 11 g fiber, 5 g sugar, 134 mg sodium
STAR NUTRIENTS: folate (39% DV), thiamin (15% DV), vitamin A (104% DV), vitamin B6 (13% DV), vitamin C (26% DV), iron (20% DV), magnesium (16% DV), potassium (21% DV)

pigeon peas with pumpkin and *sofrito*

ACTIVE PREPARATION TIME: **20 minutes** • TOTAL PREPARATION TIME: **2 hours**
(not including soaking time)

Puerto Rican cuisine boasts vibrant Latin and Caribbean flavors, with a reverent nod to local foods available on the island, such as pigeon peas and calabaza—a pumpkinlike squash commonly used in many dishes. And a Puerto Rican dish wouldn't be complete without sofrito—a traditional flavorful cooking base that includes herbs, spices, peppers, onions, and cilantro. With the help of one of my favorite tools, a pressure cooker, you can cook this up in mere minutes.

MAKES 8 SERVINGS
(1 generous cup each)

1 pound (454 g) dried pigeon peas
5 cups (1,183 ml) water, plus more for soaking
1½ pounds (680 g) calabaza (see Notes)

Sofrito
2 tablespoons extra virgin olive oil
1 tablespoon annatto seeds (see Notes)
1 medium green bell pepper, seeded and quartered
2 small sweet chile peppers, seeded and quartered
1 medium yellow onion, peeled and quartered
2 medium garlic cloves
1 cup (60 g) packed fresh cilantro sprigs
½ teaspoon dried oregano
½ cup (118 g) tomato sauce
Freshly ground black pepper, to taste
Pinch of sea salt, optional

1. Cover the pigeon peas with water and soak overnight.
2. Discard the water and place the pigeon peas in a large pot with the 5 cups of water over medium-high heat.
3. Peel the calabaza and slice it into large chunks. Add the chunks to the pot, cover, reduce the heat to medium, and simmer for about 55 minutes.
4. To make the *sofrito*: Heat the olive oil in a skillet over medium heat. Add the annatto seeds and toast for 3 to 5 minutes, until the oil turns a dark golden red. Remove the seeds with a slotted spoon and discard. Reserve the oil in the skillet.
5. Place the bell pepper, chile peppers, onion, garlic, and cilantro in a food processor. Process until finely chopped. Pour into the skillet and sauté for 10 minutes.

6. Add the oregano and tomato sauce and combine well.

7. When the beans and calabaza mixture have been cooking for one hour, add the *sofrito*. Stir well.

8. Cover and cook for an additional 50 to 60 minutes, until the consistency is thick and the beans are tender. Taste and season with black pepper and sea salt, if desired.

notes: If you cannot find calabaza, substitute kabocha squash or cooking pumpkin.

You can find annatto seeds in specialty supermarkets or online.

To prepare this dish with a pressure cooker, add the soaked beans, water, and squash to the pressure cooker and cook for 5 minutes, according to manufacturer directions. Add the *sofrito* and cook for an additional 5 minutes.

PER SERVING: 242 calories, 13 g protein, 40 g carbohydrate, 5 g fat, 1 g saturated fat, 10 g fiber, 2 g sugar, 96 mg sodium

STAR NUTRIENTS: folate (17% DV), niacin (10% DV), thiamin (27% DV), vitamin B6 (10% DV), vitamin C (29% DV), iron (19% DV), magnesium (28% DV), manganese (17% DV), potassium (26% DV), zinc (11% DV)

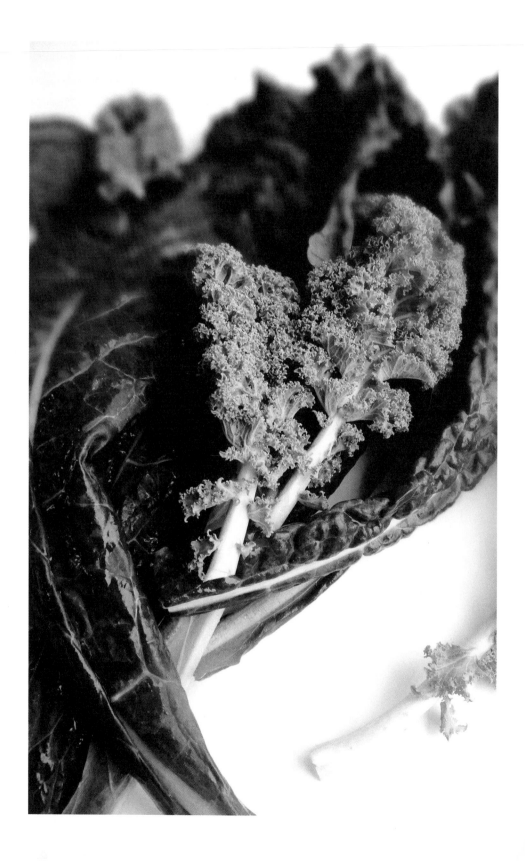

Lose your fear of fats.

Fresh Guacamole with Tomatoes and Serrano Chiles
Pecan-Cherry-Chia Nutrition Bars

few decades ago, we were smack in the middle of the fat-phobia era. It started when scientists learned that saturated fats in the diet raised cholesterol levels, which are linked to heart disease. But instead of preaching the low-saturated-fat message, health experts simplified it to the low-fat message. In response, food manufacturers started stripping fat from foods and plastering "fat-free" and "low-fat" claims on food labels. Unfortunately, they replaced the fat with refined carbs, such as sugar and white flour, to make them palatable.

Now we know that we threw the baby out with the bathwater. Sure enough, you should still keep your saturated fat intake to a minimum—less than 10 percent of your daily calories (about 20 grams for the average person). In addition, artificial trans fat—found in partially hydrogenated vegetable oils used in processed foods like margarine, popcorn, and fried foods—is even worse for your heart and should be avoided altogether. (As of this writing, the FDA is moving to ban trans fats in the United States.) But some fats are actually *good* for your heart: monounsaturated and polyunsaturated fats.

It's just another sign of the benefits of a plant-based diet: plant-based fats, such as nuts, seeds, olives, avocados, and vegetable oils, tend to be low in saturated fat and rich in heart-healthy monounsaturated and polyunsaturated fats. Try to include a small amount of these foods in your diet every day. There is one exception: tropical oils, such as palm kernel oil, palm oil, and coconut oil, are high in saturated fat. Palm oil is increasingly popular as a food ingredient used by food manufacturers, and much hype has been made over coconut oil's potential health benefits. However, there is not enough research to prove purported benefits, such as weight loss or brain protection, for these types of fat, and they are not as heart healthy as unsaturated vegetable oils such as extra virgin olive oil. My suggestion is to enjoy small amounts of tropical nuts as part of your saturated fat budget, such as coconut milk in a curry (see page 144), but don't switch to their oils in an attempt to gain better health.

Regardless of oil choice, remember that fat is a concentrated source of calories—a little goes a long way. Limit your servings to a handful of nuts, a couple of tablespoonfuls of seeds, and one eighth of an avocado. And when you use vegetable oils, such as extra virgin olive oil, in salad dressings, side dishes, and entrées, use just a drizzle to add wonderful flavor and healthy fats.

fresh guacamole with tomatoes and serrano chiles

ACTIVE PREPARATION TIME: **10 minutes** • TOTAL PREPARATION TIME: **10 minutes**

I am lucky enough to have a half century-old avocado tree growing in front of my house that produces hundreds of rich, creamy avocados each year. But even without your own tree, avocados are worth seeking out—packed with healthy monounsaturated fats, as well as antioxidant phytochemicals, they're great for helping to keep your heart ticking smoothly. This flavorful guacamole goes well with tortilla chips or veggies, or as an accompaniment for Latin dishes, such as Pinto Bean and Tofu Breakfast Rancheros (page 136).

MAKES 10 SERVINGS
(about 3 tablespoons each)

2 medium ripe avocados, halved, pitted, and peeled
3 medium garlic cloves, minced
Juice of 1 medium lemon
½ small serrano chile, seeded and finely diced
1 tablespoon chopped fresh cilantro leaves
¼ cup (37 g) quartered grape tomatoes or small cherry tomatoes
Dash of salt, optional

1. In a small bowl, mash the avocados with a fork or potato masher until smooth yet somewhat lumpy.
2. Add the garlic, lemon juice, serrano chile, cilantro, and tomatoes and mix well.
3. Taste and season with salt, if desired. Serve immediately.

note: To adjust the spiciness, use more or less of the serrano chile.

You may store the guacamole in an airtight container in the refrigerator for up to 2 days, although the color may dull slightly.

variations: Substitute another chile pepper, such as Anaheim, jalapeño, or habanero; substitute lime juice for lemon juice.

PER SERVING: 51 calories, 1 g protein, 4 g carbohydrate, 4 g fat, .5 g saturated fat, 2 g fiber, 1 g sugar, 3 mg sodium
STAR NUTRIENTS: vitamin C (25% DV)

pecan-cherry-chia nutrition bars

ACTIVE PREPARATION TIME: **14 minutes** • TOTAL PREPARATION TIME: **14 minutes**
(not including chilling time)

Don't shy away from nuts and seeds just because they have rich supplies of fat. Remember, these are heart-healthy plant-based fats, so let them star in these homemade nutrition bars. Who needs to buy prefabricated granola bars when you can make a batch of these naturally sweet goodies in minutes—no baking required? Sweetened with dried cherries and raisins, these bars are packed with wholesome goodness, thanks to an all-star lineup of pecans, oats, whole grains, coconut, chia, sunflower seeds, and cinnamon. Pack them in your gym, lunch, or travel bag, as well as your kids' backpacks. You can even change up the ingredients to use your favorite fruits, seeds, and nuts. Get in the homemade nutrition bar game today!

MAKES 16 SERVINGS
(1 bar each)

½ cup (82 g) finely chopped dried cherries (see Notes)
¼ cup (41 g) finely chopped raisins (see Notes)
½ cup (55 g) chopped pecans
¾ cup (117 g) old-fashioned oats
¾ cup (30 g) unsweetened whole grain flaked cold breakfast
    cereal, such as wheat or buckwheat
1½ tablespoons shredded unsweetened coconut
1½ tablespoons chia seeds
½ cup (128 g) sunflower seed butter
¼ cup (85 g) honey or agave nectar
3 tablespoons water
½ teaspoon vanilla extract
½ teaspoon cinnamon

1. Line a 9-inch square dish with plastic wrap, leaving enough extra to cover the top of the dish later.
2. Mix together the cherries, raisins, pecans, oats, cereal, coconut, and chia seeds in a medium bowl.
3. Combine the sunflower seed butter, honey, and water in a small pot over medium heat and cook, stirring, for 2 minutes, until thin and smooth. Remove from the heat and stir in the vanilla and cinnamon until well blended.
4. Stir the sunflower seed butter mixture into the fruit mixture. Mix with clean hands to distribute all ingredients.

5. Transfer the mixture into the lined dish and pat down firmly. Cover with plastic wrap and refrigerate at least 3 hours, until firm.

6. Slice into 16 bars. Store in an airtight container in the refrigerator.

notes: These bars freeze well. Wrap them individually in plastic wrap for convenient snacks.

Don't skip chopping the raisins; it's necessary to hold the bars together.

Neither the raisins nor the cherries should be packed when measured out.

variations: You may substitute chopped apricots for the cherries; peanut or almond butter for the sunflower seed butter; and walnuts, hazelnuts, peanuts, or macadamia nuts for the pecans. To make this gluten-free, use gluten-free oats and breakfast cereal flakes, and check that the nuts and seeds are gluten-free.

PER SERVING: 136 calories, 3 g protein, 17 g carbohydrate, 8 g fat, 1 g saturated fat, 2 g fiber, 10 g sugar, 13 mg sodium

STAR NUTRIENTS: folate (16% DV), niacin (10% DV), vitamin B6 (10% DV), vitamin C (10% DV), vitamin E (14% DV), iron (11% DV), manganese (17% DV), zinc (10% DV)

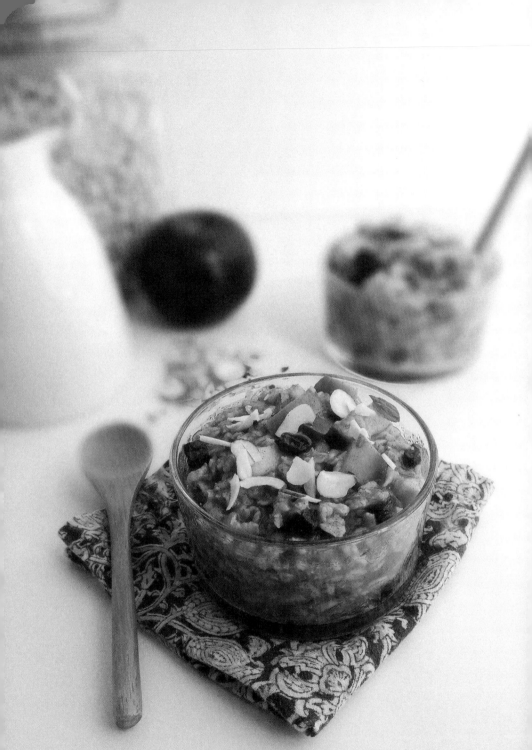

Scandinavian Apple-Cardamom Oatmeal

Power up on nuts and seeds.

Seeded Whole Wheat Biscuits
Scandinavian Apple-Cardamom Oatmeal
Artisanal Nut and Seed Spread

N uts and seeds aren't just for squirrels; they're ideal nutrition for you, too. These tiny kernels are packed with potent nutrients, such as protein (up to 9 grams per 1-ounce serving!), fiber, healthy fats, vitamins, minerals, and phytochemicals. A body of research shows that eating about one to two ounces of nuts (walnuts, pecans, almonds, pistachios, macadamia nuts, Brazil nuts, hazelnuts, or cashews) or peanuts (botanically a legume, but similar in nutrition profile to nuts) daily can grant protection against heart disease, type 2 diabetes, and some types of cancer. Nuts have also been linked to better brain function, weight control, and improved fertility.

Seeds, such as sesame, sunflower, pumpkin, hemp, and chia, may not have garnered as much research on health benefits as have nuts, but they too are rich sources of healthy fats, protein, fiber, vitamins, minerals, and phytochemicals.

Some nuts and seeds—such as walnuts, hemp, chia, and flax—are rich sources of heart- and brain-friendly omega-3 fatty acids. Other nuts are rich in specific nutrients: almonds in calcium, sunflower seeds in vitamin E. So, boost your diet every day with the plant protein and potent nutrients found in one to two servings (one ounce of nuts or seeds, or two tablespoons of nut or seed butter) of a variety of nuts and seeds. It's easy: just sprinkle flax (ground, so you can absorb its nutrients), hemp, or chia into cereals and smoothies; stir chopped nuts into porridge; spread nut or seed butters over whole grain toast or flatbread; sprinkle nuts or seeds over salads; and fold nuts, seeds, and their butters into baked goods, such as bars, breads, and muffins. Best of all, whether you're on the run or relaxing at home, a handful of nuts or seeds makes for one of the best snacks on the planet.

seeded whole wheat biscuits

ACTIVE PREPARATION TIME: **10 minutes** • TOTAL PREPARATION TIME: **30 minutes**

Nuts and seeds may make for a nutritious snack, but you can also harness their power in creative ways, such as these wholesome biscuits. There's nothing like the aroma and flavor of a tender, flaky biscuit, hot out of the oven. And you don't have to miss out on whole grains, either: each biscuit is packed with whole wheat, as well as sesame, hemp, and flaxseeds for a heart-healthy nutritional profile and a flavorful crunch. Serve these biscuits for breakfast slathered with nut butter and fruit spread, or at lunch or dinner with a soup, chili, or bean stew, such as Caribbean Calypso Beans (page 24).

MAKES 10 SERVINGS
(1 biscuit each)

1¾ cups (210 g) whole wheat pastry flour
1 tablespoon ground flaxseeds
1 tablespoon sesame seeds
1 tablespoon hemp seeds
1 tablespoon baking powder
⅓ cup (75 g) soft dairy-free margarine (see Notes on page 223)
¾ cup (178 ml) unsweetened plain plant-based milk

1. Preheat the oven to 375°F (190°C).
2. Mix together the flour, flaxseeds, sesame seeds, hemp seeds, and baking powder.
3. Cut in the margarine with a fork.
4. Stir in the plant-based milk to form a stiff dough.
5. Roll out onto a lightly floured surface to a 1½-inch thickness.
6. Using a 2½-inch round cutter (or inverted drinking glass), cut out 10 biscuits.
7. Place the biscuits on a baking sheet and bake for about 20 minutes, until lightly browned on the surface.

variations: Substitute finely chopped sunflower seeds or pumpkin seeds for the sesame seeds. For a gluten-free version, substitute a gluten-free flour blend (e.g., Bob's Red Mill or King Arthur Flour) for the whole wheat pastry flour and check that all other ingredients are gluten-free.

PER SERVING: 120 calories, 4 g protein, 16 g carbohydrate, 5 g fat, 1 g saturated fat, 3 g fiber, 0 g sugar, 95 mg sodium
STAR NUTRIENTS: thiamin (10% DV), calcium (11% DV), phosphorus (12% DV)

See photo
on page 208

scandinavian apple-cardamom oatmeal

ACTIVE PREPARATION TIME: **5 minutes** • TOTAL PREPARATION TIME: **13 minutes**

A sprinkling of nuts at breakfast time can power your day with a punch of protein, healthy fats, fiber, and more. Nuts or seeds are the perfect partner for hot cereals, along with a serving of fruit and splash of plant-based milk. It's hard to find a better start to your day! And this hearty porridge is inspired by the traditional flavors—oats, apples, almonds, cardamom—of Sweden, where gröt (Swedish for porridge) is a classic start of the day for both children and adults alike. Quick, nutritious, and delicious, this recipe will please the palates of everyone in the family.

MAKES 2 SERVINGS
(about 1¼ cups each)

2¼ cups (532 ml) water
1 cup (156 g) uncooked old-fashioned oats
1 medium apple, diced
3 tablespoons dried currants or raisins
1 tablespoon agave nectar or honey, optional
½ teaspoon ground cardamom
3 tablespoons sliced almonds
Plant-based milk, optional

1. Bring the water to a boil in a medium saucepan over high heat.
2. Add the oats, apple, currants, agave (if desired), and cardamom and stir well. Cover and reduce the heat to medium. Cook for 8 minutes, stirring occasionally, until apple is tender.
3. Stir in the almonds and serve immediately with plant-based milk, if desired.

note: You can make a double batch of this recipe, store it in an airtight container in the refrigerator for up to 3 days, and microwave it each morning for an easy meal solution. In that case, add the almonds right before serving to retain their crunch.

PER SERVING: 214 calories, 5 g protein, 39 g carbohydrate, 6 g fat, .5 g saturated fat, 6 g fiber, 18 g sugar, 6 mg sodium
STAR NUTRIENTS: riboflavin (15% DV), vitamin C (12% DV), vitamin E (12% DV), iron (14% DV), manganese (10% DV)

artisanal nut and seed spread

ACTIVE PREPARATION TIME: **10 minutes** • TOTAL PREPARATION TIME: **10 minutes**

Nut and seed butters are a popular way to enjoy the protein, healthy fats, fiber, and antioxidants of these plant foods. But did you know that you can make your own artisanal brand of nut or seed butter at home—just the way you like it? This version is loaded with a variety of nuts and seeds, as well as cocoa powder, cinnamon, and a touch of sweetness. Blend up a batch and use it on your whole grain toast, sandwiches, or crudités all week long.

MAKES 8 SERVINGS
(about 1½ tablespoons each)

¼ cup (37 g) unsalted whole peanuts
¼ cup (35 g) unsalted whole almonds
¼ cup (25 g) unsalted whole pecans
1 tablespoon whole flaxseeds
1 tablespoon hemp seeds
1 tablespoon unsalted sunflower seeds
2 tablespoons peanut oil
1 tablespoon cocoa powder
½ teaspoon cinnamon
1 teaspoon honey or maple syrup

1. Combine all the ingredients in a small food processor or blender. Process for about 3 to 5 minutes into a spreadable yet chunky consistency. Pause and scrape down the sides of the blender as needed.

note: Store in an airtight container at room temperature for up to 3 weeks.

variations: You may substitute unsalted hazelnuts, walnuts, pine nuts, or pistachios for the peanuts, almonds, or pecans. You may also substitute chia or sesame seeds for the hemp seeds.

PER SERVING: 157 calories, 4 g protein, 5 g carbohydrate, 15 g fat, 1.5 g saturated fat, 2 g fiber, 1.5 g sugar, 1 mg sodium
STAR NUTRIENTS: vitamin E (11% DV), magnesium (10% DV), manganese (29% DV)

Ginger-Cardamom
Baked Acorn Squash

Honor the growing seasons of plants.

Creamed Spring Peas and Potatoes
Ginger-Cardamom Baked Acorn Squash
Stone Fruit Trifle

Nature is a delicious cycle. As spring's first tentative warm rays come, the soil thaws, seeds sprout, and tender shoots greet the sun. And as the days become warmer, plants mature and produce leaves, fruits, and seeds— the source of food for humans. As the sunny days ebb into autumn, they wait for their annual renewal in the spring. Our ancestors understood this cycle as surely as they knew to build a fire for warmth and to seek shelter for protection. They gathered nature's abundance in the spring, summer, and fall, and stored it away for the winter—in root cellars, grain bags, and earthenware jars. But today, how many people know when the growing season is for blueberries, lettuce, or pears? Just walk down a supermarket produce aisle and you can find all three every day of the year.

What's wrong with eating anything we want, anytime we want it? Well, first of all, in order to have fresh produce year-round, it's often grown in faraway locations with opposite or longer growing seasons, or in a greenhouse, heated to a cozy temperature, compliments of fossil fuels. Then, that out-of-season produce is transported for long distances, burning up lots of fuel along the way to your shopping cart. To top it off, foods are often picked green in order to make the long trip without going bad. Less mature foods may not contain the same quality of nutrition or flavor as foods picked in their ripe perfection.

I'm not saying that you should never eat lettuce in December—I do, myself— but there is much to be gained by acknowledging the natural growing seasons of plants. Enjoy the best of summer's fresh fruits and vegetables—apricots, peaches, watermelon, green beans, zucchini—especially those grown in your local community. And during late fall and winter, feast on cool-weather produce—plants harvested later in the year that have a long shelf life—such as apples, potatoes, carrots, turnips, and winter squash. A good seasonal guide for fresh produce is available on my website, sharonpalmer.com, or at USDA.gov.

Eat, breathe, and live with the seasons.

creamed spring peas and potatoes

ACTIVE PREPARATION TIME: **10 minutes** • TOTAL PREPARATION TIME: **28 minutes**

My mother would make this every time she harvested fresh peas and new potatoes from our kitchen garden. This dish—one of the first prizes from her garden—heralded the arrival of spring. It's such a simple side dish that showcases the flavors of farm-fresh produce, whether you acquire it from your own garden, local supermarket, farmers market or CSA.

MAKES 6 SERVINGS
(½ cup each)

1 cup (150 g) sliced fingerling potatoes, with skins
3 cups (711 ml) water
10 ounces (283 g) shelled fresh peas (see Notes)
1 teaspoon extra virgin olive oil
1 small garlic clove, minced
2 teaspoons chopped fresh dill, or ½ teaspoon dried
Pinch of freshly ground black pepper
Pinch of sea salt, optional
1 tablespoon plus 1 teaspoon flour (see Notes)
1 cup (237 ml) unsweetened plain plant-based milk

1. Place the potatoes and water in a medium pot over medium-high heat, cover, and bring to a boil. Reduce heat to medium and boil for 8 minutes. Add the peas, cover, and cook for about 7 additional minutes, until the potatoes are tender when pierced with a fork (do not overcook—the peas should be bright green and solid).

2. Meanwhile, heat the olive oil in a sauté pan. Add the garlic, dill, black pepper, and sea salt, if desired, and sauté, stirring, for 3 minutes. Add the flour and stir for 15 seconds to make a paste, then stir in the plant-based milk with a wire whisk. Heat until thickened and bubbly, about 2 minutes. Remove from the heat.

3. Drain the cooked vegetables and stir in the sauce. Serve immediately.

notes: You may substitute frozen peas for fresh if they aren't in season.

You may substitute 2 teaspoons cornstarch for the flour to make this dish gluten-free. If you do, mix the cornstarch into the plant-based milk in step 2.

PER SERVING: 83 calories, 4 g protein, 13 g carbohydrate, 2 g fat, 0 g saturated fat, 3 g fiber, 3 g sugar, 74 mg sodium
STAR NUTRIENTS: folate (11% DV), thiamin (11% DV), vitamin C (40% DV), vitamin K (16% DV)

ginger-cardamom baked acorn squash

See photo
on page 214

I love when the warm weather gives way to the cool, crisp days of fall and the winter squashes start to appear in supermarkets and farmers markets. Winter squashes, which can last for weeks in your kitchen, are also rich in the heart-loving nutrient beta-carotene. This sweet and flavorful recipe is so simple—just split open a small squash, scoop out the seeds, and season it with ginger, spices, and almonds. And it will fill your kitchen with wonderful aromas!

MAKES 4 SERVINGS
(¼ squash)

One 4-inch-diameter (431 g) acorn squash
Juice of ½ lemon
1½ teaspoons extra virgin olive oil
1 teaspoon honey or agave nectar
1 teaspoon crystallized ginger, mashed with a mortar and pestle
¼ teaspoon turmeric
¼ teaspoon cardamom
2 tablespoons slivered almonds

1. Preheat the oven to 350°F (180°C).
2. Split the squash in half and scoop out the seeds. Place in a baking dish, cavity side facing up, and cover the bottom of the dish with ½ inch of water.
3. Mix together the lemon juice, olive oil, honey, crystallized ginger, turmeric, and cardamom in a small dish. Drizzle half of the mixture evenly over each squash half.
4. Sprinkle the slivered almonds on top of the squash halves.
5. Place the dish in the oven and bake until the squash is golden and tender, about 45 minutes.

variation: Use any small squash for this recipe, such as butternut, buttercup, or kabocha.

PER SERVING: 114 calories, 2 g protein, 20 g carbohydrate, 4.5 g fat, .5 g saturated fat, 6 g fiber, 7 g sugar, 5 mg sodium
STAR NUTRIENTS: thiamin (29% DV), vitamin A (32% DV), vitamin B6 (11% DV), vitamin C (37% DV), magnesium (15% DV), potassium (15% DV)

stone fruit trifle

A traditional English trifle has thick layers of cream, cake, and fruit, which meld together to create a truly delectable flavor and texture. This healthy plant-powered version calls upon this tradition in order to provide a cool, creamy summertime treat you can indulge in any day of the week. It's a perfect recipe to showcase a summer trip to the farmers market, when ripe stone fruit—peaches, apricots, and plums—are in season.

MAKES 10 SERVINGS
(about ⅔ cup each)

2 tablespoons sliced almonds
Two 6-ounce (170 g) cartons Greek-style vanilla coconut yogurt
2 tablespoons sherry, optional
¾ cup (240 g) unsweetened raspberry fruit spread
One 8-ounce (227 g) package graham cracker sticks (gluten-free, if desired; see Notes)
5 fresh apricots, sliced
3 fresh plums, sliced
2 medium fresh peaches, peeled, if desired, and sliced

1. Preheat the oven to 350°F (180°C).
2. Place the almonds in a small dish and toast in the oven for about 5 minutes, until golden. Remove and let cool.
3. Pour the yogurt into a small mixing bowl and beat with a spoon for a minute, until smooth and creamy.
4. If using the sherry, mix with the raspberry fruit spread in a small dish until smooth.
5. To make the trifle, select a medium glass bowl (see Notes). Layer as follows: one third of the graham cracker sticks, one third of the yogurt, one third of the raspberry fruit spread, all of the apricots, one third of the graham cracker sticks, one third of the yogurt, one third of the raspberry fruit spread, all of the plums, the remaining graham cracker sticks, the remaining coconut yogurt, the remaining raspberry fruit spread, and all of the peaches. Sprinkle the toasted almonds on top.
6. Cover the trifle and refrigerate for about 1 hour. Spoon into dishes to serve.

notes: Back to Nature Graham Cracker Sticks are a good option; if using gluten-free crackers, I recommend Schar Gluten-Free Honeygrams (you'll need to break them into "sticks" yourself).

A trifle dish is perfect for this recipe, because the bottom of the dish is the same size as the top. If you use a rounded bowl, your bottom layer will be thicker than the other layers. While this recipe benefits from chilling for about 1 hour prior to serving to allow flavors to meld, it does not keep well. Try to enjoy it within 8 hours of preparation.

PER SERVING: 174 calories, 3 g protein, 35 g carbohydrate, 4.5 g fat, 2 g saturated fat, 2 g fiber, 17 g sugar, 133 mg sodium
STAR NUTRIENTS: vitamin A (25% DV), vitamin C (23% DV), manganese (21% DV)

Creamy Peanut Butter Pie

Enjoy sweets—when they're worth it.

Creamy Peanut Butter Pie

Applesauce Raisin Snack Cake

Sweet Potato and Pecan Maple Pie

Thanks to the availability of processed convenience foods, our sweet tooth has really flourished. I remember as a child a sweet treat was just that: a treat. I really looked forward to that thick, frosted cake on my birthday, the fresh fruit pies my mom made for summer family reunions, and Christmas, when a flurry of holiday cookies graced the kitchen countertop. But these foods were hardly routine.

Over the years, our sugar intake has steadily increased—we consumed on average 19 percent more between 1970 and 2005. That's because you don't have to wait for Mom to bake that apple pie or batch of chocolate chip cookies anymore—you can pick up these goodies anywhere. While it's great to enjoy delicious, traditional foods—even desserts—it's best to keep treats to a minimum. Our high intake of added sugars has been linked with weight gain, metabolic problems, and heart risk.

So, here's my advice on doing sweets right. Your finale at most meals should be nutrient-packed fruit—nature's own dessert. These naturally sweet gems come packed with fiber, vitamins, minerals, and disease-fighting compounds. The second runner-up to fruit should be lightly sweetened, nutrient-rich, whole plant foods–based desserts, such as fruit cobbler (see Peach and Cranberry Crumble, page 107) or a whole grain treat (see Applesauce Raisin Snack Cake, page 224). And then for those special occasions, go ahead and indulge in a slice of cake or a pastry.

In fact, it's okay to enjoy a small indulgence—an ounce of dark chocolate, a small whole grain fruit bar (see page 206)—every day, as long as you keep the portion reasonable and within your energy needs. Just remember to make these treats worthwhile by focusing on quality ingredients, such as dark chocolate, spices, and fruits, rather than highly processed ingredients, like hydrogenated oils, high-fructose corn syrup, and preservatives. Most importantly, savor the flavors and really *enjoy* your treat.

See photo
on page 220

creamy peanut butter pie

ACTIVE PREPARATION TIME: **22 minutes** • TOTAL PREPARATION TIME: **27 minutes**
(not including chilling time)

You won't believe that this light and luscious pie—kissed with the dynamic duo of peanut butter and dark chocolate—is made with tofu and only a touch of agave nectar for sweetness. In fact, this is a nutrient-rich dessert you can really feel good about indulging in!

MAKES 8 SERVINGS
(one-eighth pie each)

Graham Cracker Crust
22 graham cracker halves (whole wheat or gluten-free, if de-
    sired—see Notes on page 219)
½ teaspoon cinnamon
2 tablespoons wheat germ or ground flaxseeds
¼ cup (56 g) melted soft dairy-free margarine (see Notes)

Filling
One 12.3-ounce (349 g) package extra firm silken tofu
1 cup (258 g) unsalted creamy peanut butter
1½ teaspoons vanilla extract
5 tablespoons agave nectar
2 tablespoons unsweetened plain plant-based milk

Garnish
⅓ cup (45 g) dairy-free dark chocolate chips (see Notes)
2 tablespoons chopped peanuts

1. Preheat the oven to 375°F (180°C).
2. Add the graham crackers to a blender in batches and pulse into crumbs, or crush into crumbs using a rolling pin.
3. Mix the graham cracker crumbs, cinnamon, and wheat germ in a medium bowl. Stir in the melted margarine.
4. Press the crumb mixture into a 9-inch pie pan. Bake for 10 to 12 minutes. Remove the crust from the oven and set it aside to cool.
5. Meanwhile, place the tofu, peanut butter, vanilla, agave, and plant-based milk in a large mixing bowl. Beat with an electric mixer until smooth, fluffy, and creamy, scraping down the sides of the bowl as needed.
6. Place the dark chocolate chips into a small, microwave-proof dish and microwave on high for 2 minutes. Stir the chocolate with a spoon until smooth.

7. Pour the tofu filling evenly into the cooled graham cracker crust.

8. Drizzle the chocolate over the top of the pie. Sprinkle with the chopped peanuts. Chill for 2 hours before slicing.

notes: Choose a dairy-free margarine that comes in a tub, not in sticks. Earth Balance is one good option, but there are other brands that also have a good low saturated fat profile.

You may also use chopped dairy-free dark chocolate instead of chocolate chips.

variation: Stir one sliced banana into the filling before step 7 to make Peanut Butter Banana Pie.

PER SERVING: 374 calories, 12 g protein, 25 g carbohydrate, 27 g fat, 6 g saturated fat, 4 g fiber, 11 g sugar, 134 mg sodium

STAR NUTRIENTS: folate (14% DV), niacin (27% DV), vitamin B6 (11% DV), vitamin E (19% DV), iron (13% DV), magnesium (19% DV), manganese (17% DV), potassium (10% DV), zinc (11% DV)

---

applesauce raisin snack cake

This moist, delicious whole grain cake—which garners its sweetness from applesauce and raisins—is healthy enough to pack along in your lunch bag or to serve as an after-school snack to a hungry pack of kids. Pop extra slices in the freezer to pull out later when you're in the mood for a sweet bite.

MAKES 16 SERVINGS
(one-sixteenth cake each)

½ cup (83 g) raisins
½ cup hot water
Nonstick cooking spray
1 cup (244 g) unsweetened applesauce (homemade, if desired; see page 343)
¼ cup (59 ml) canola oil, expeller pressed
3 tablespoons agave nectar
2 tablespoons chia seeds (see Notes on page 139)
2 cups (240 g) white whole wheat flour
2 teaspoons baking powder
½ teaspoon baking soda
1 teaspoon cinnamon
¼ teaspoon nutmeg
¼ teaspoon cloves
⅓ cup (44 g) chopped walnuts
¼ cup (30 g) dairy-free dark chocolate chips

1. Combine the raisins and hot water in a small dish and set aside for 5 minutes to soften.

2. Preheat the oven to 350°F (180°C). Spray a 9 by 9-inch baking pan with nonstick cooking spray.

3. In a mixing bowl, combine the applesauce, canola oil, agave, and chia seeds and beat well with a wire whisk or an electric mixer for 2 minutes. Add the softened raisins and their soaking liquid and combine well.

4. Stir in the flour, baking powder, baking soda, cinnamon, nutmeg, cloves, and walnuts, just until combined (do not overmix).

5. Pour the batter into the pan. Sprinkle with the chocolate chips.

6. Bake for 25 to 30 minutes, until a fork inserted into the center of the cake comes out clean. Let the cake cool slightly and cut into 16 squares.

note: This cake is great served immediately while warm. Freeze leftover slices in an airtight container for up to one month.

variation: To make gluten-free, substitute 1½ cups all-purpose gluten-free flour blend (such as Bob's Red Mill or King Arthur Flour) for the 2 cups white whole wheat flour and check that all other ingredients are gluten-free.

PER SERVING: 152 calories, 3 g protein, 23 g carbohydrate, 7 g fat, 1 g saturated fat, 3 g fiber, 8 g sugar, 42 mg sodium
STAR NUTRIENTS: manganese (40% DV), phosphorus (13% DV), selenium (15% DV)

sweet potato and pecan maple pie

ACTIVE PREPARATION TIME: **28 minutes** • TOTAL PREPARATION TIME: **1 hour 25 minutes**

This rich, nutty pie is perfect for a holiday, such as Thanksgiving or Christmas. You won't believe that this dairy-free pie with a whole grain crust is sweetened with only a touch of maple syrup. And it's just as good the next day.

MAKES 10 SERVINGS
(one-tenth pie each)

2 large (567 g) sweet potatoes, peeled and coarsely chopped
3 cups (711 ml) plus 5 to 6 tablespoons water
1½ cups (180 g) whole wheat pastry flour
½ cup (56 g) pecan meal (see Note)
5 tablespoons soft dairy-free margarine (see Notes on page 223)
¼ cup plus 1 teaspoon (88 g) maple syrup
1 cup (237 ml) vanilla plant-based milk
2 tablespoons cornstarch
¼ teaspoon cloves
¼ teaspoon nutmeg
¼ teaspoon allspice
1¼ teaspoons cinnamon
½ cup (55 g) coarsely chopped pecans

1. Preheat the oven to 375°F (190°C).
2. Place the sweet potatoes in a medium pot and cover with the 3 cups (711 ml) of water. Cover with a lid and boil over medium heat for about 20 minutes, until the sweet potatoes are tender. Drain well, return the sweet potatoes to the pot and mash with a potato masher to form a smooth mixture, and set aside.
3. Meanwhile, mix together the whole wheat pastry flour and pecan meal in a small bowl. Cut in the margarine using a fork or a pastry cutter until crumbly. Add the water, 1 tablespoon at a time, and mix with a wooden spoon into a stiff dough. On a lightly floured surface, roll the dough out to fit a 9-inch pie pan. Place the piecrust into the pan; you may need to shape and press it into the pan with your fingers. Score with a fork. Bake for 10 minutes. Remove from oven.
4. To make the filling, add ¼ cup maple syrup to the pot with the mashed sweet potatoes. Mix together the plant-based milk and cornstarch until smooth and add to the pot. Add the cloves, nutmeg, allspice, and 1 teaspoon of the cinnamon and stir to combine well. Heat the contents, stirring constantly with a wire whisk, until thick and bubbly (about 2 minutes).

5. Pour the filling into the partially baked pie shell and place in the oven at 375°F (190°C). Bake for 45 minutes.

6. Mix the pecans, remaining 1 teaspoon maple syrup, and remaining ¼ teaspoon cinnamon. Sprinkle over the pie and return it to the oven for an additional 10 minutes.

7. Cool slightly before serving.

note: You can find pecan meal at natural and online food purveyors (such as Bob's Red Mill). You also can substitute almond or peanut meal or flour for pecan meal.

variation: To make this gluten-free, substitute 1¼ cups all-purpose gluten-free flour blend (such as Bob's Red Mill or King Arthur Flour) for the 1½ cups whole wheat pastry flour and check that all other ingredients are gluten-free.

PER SERVING: 292 calories, 4 g protein, 45 g carbohydrate, 11 g fat, 1 g saturated fat, 4 g fiber, 23 g sugar, 75 mg sodium
STAR NUTRIENTS: riboflavin (31% DV), vitamin A (143% DV), vitamin C (12% DV), manganese (35% DV)

Eat the whole plant.

Lentils with Wild Mushrooms and Broccoli Rabe
Borscht with Beets and Beet Greens

D o you peel away the skins of carrots and lop off the tops of your beets? If the answer is yes, you might want to rethink this practice. You see, plants did something really smart in their quest for survival. They deposited high levels of their nutrients and phytochemicals in their outer coverings or skins for protection against predators (see page 000). And in their seeds, they developed fiber-rich, protective coatings, packed with healthy oils and antioxidants inside, to ensure the survival of the new plant when it sprouted from the seed. The plant's green leaves were packed with chlorophyll, which traps light energy and produces food for the plant, along with dozens of essential vitamins and minerals for humans. And below the ground, tuberous and swollen roots formed, storing energy and nutrients to feed the shoots of a new plant. These parts offered sustenance—and protection—for the plant to grow and prosper.

All of these edible components of the plant have been a vital source of nutrients for humans throughout history. But today we often cast away the most nutrient-rich parts of plants—outer coverings, seeds, leaves—in search for the starchiest, sweetest section in the middle. While it's true that not every edible plant can be eaten in its entirety, many may be consumed skins, flesh, seeds, leaves, and all! Beets, carrots, and turnips are but a few examples of plants that can be savored root to stem. One habit worth instilling is to preserve the peels of plants as much as possible. Don't peel away the nutrients found in cucumber, potato, apple, pear, and carrot skins. For many of these foods, you can give the outer skin a good scrubbing and you're good to go. Choose foods that possess their skins intact, such as whole grains, beans, lentils, peas, fruits, bell peppers, eggplants, and chia seeds. And don't miss out on the beauty of the whole plant by opting for juices, which don't include the fibrous pulps, seeds, and peels of fruits and vegetables. Keep it simple—eat the whole plant and nothing but the plant.

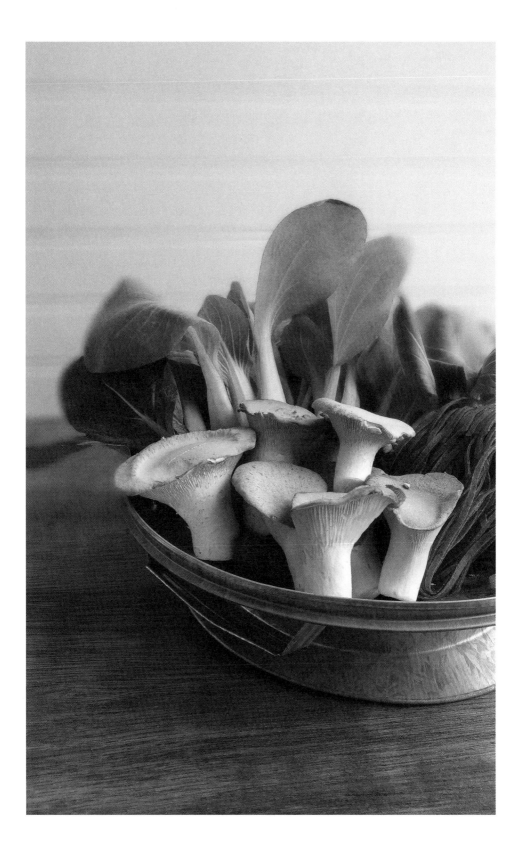

lentils with wild mushrooms
and broccoli rabe

ACTIVE PREPARATION TIME: **10 minutes** • TOTAL PREPARATION TIME: **39 minutes**

It's hard to get more "whole" than this dish, featuring broccoli rabe—a green, nutrient-packed vegetable that you eat leaves, stems, buds, and all. Served with earthy lentils, this dish provides a great source of plant proteins, fiber, vitamins, and minerals that can help you fight chronic disease. Add a bright salad, such as Kiwi Herb Salad with Pistachios and Orange Dressing (page 302), to round out your meal.

MAKES 6 SERVINGS
(about 1⅓ cups each)

1 tablespoon plus 1 teaspoon extra virgin olive oil
1 medium onion, diced
2 medium garlic cloves, minced
Pinch of freshly ground black pepper
1 teaspoon dried thyme
1 teaspoon low-sodium herbal seasoning blend (see page 345)
1 tablespoon balsamic vinegar
4 cups plus 3 tablespoons (992 ml) water
2 teaspoons reduced sodium vegetable broth base
2 cups (384 g) dried green lentils
½ cup (15 g) dried wild mushrooms
One bunch broccoli rabe (about 1 pound/454 g), coarsely
    chopped (see Note)

1. Heat 1 tablespoon of the olive oil in a sauté pan over medium heat. Add the onions and sauté for 6 minutes.
2. Add the garlic, black pepper, thyme, herbal seasoning, and vinegar and stir for an additional minute.
3. Combine 4 cups of the water and broth base in a large pot. Cover and bring to a boil over high heat.
4. Transfer the onion mixture to the pot of boiling water and set the sauté pan aside for later, with juices reserved. Add the lentils and mushrooms to the pot, cover, and reduce the heat to medium. Cook for about 20 minutes, until the lentils are tender but intact.
5. About 6 minutes before the lentils are done, heat the remaining 1 teaspoon of olive oil and 3 tablespoons water in the used sauté pan over medium-high heat. Add the broccoli rabe, cover, and cook for 5 to 6 minutes, until crisp-tender and bright green.

6. To serve, place the lentils on a platter and arrange the broccoli rabe on top.

note: Broccoli rabe is also known as rapini or broccoli raab. You may substitute young stem broccoli or broccolini for broccoli rabe, if not available.

PER SERVING: 331 calories, 19 g protein, 57 g carbohydrates, 4 g fat, .5 g saturated fat, 23 g fiber, 4 g sugar, 15 mg sodium

STAR NUTRIENTS: folate (95% DV), niacin (23% DV), riboflavin (26% DV), thiamin (40% DV), vitamin A (13% DV), vitamin B6 (29% DV), vitamin C (26% DV), vitamin K (234% DV), iron (32% DV), magnesium (29% DV), manganese (17% DV), phosphorus (12% DV), potassium (30% DV), zinc (31% DV)

borscht with beets and beet greens

ACTIVE PREPARATION TIME: **19 minutes** • TOTAL PREPARATION TIME: **41 minutes**

Even in cold climates, people have long found ways to cultivate and celebrate vegetables, realizing their importance for health and sustenance. This humble Eastern European dish is based on rugged beets and cabbage. In my version, I include one of the most nutritious parts of the beet—the greens—to add a touch of pungent, green flavor. This fuchsia-colored soup, packed with powerful phytochemicals, is the perfect wintertime accompaniment to a toasted sandwich, veggie burger, or wrap. And take a lesson from this recipe—don't toss out the beet greens! They offer a savory-bitter flavor and powerful nutrition to your meals.

MAKE 8 SERVINGS
(about 1¼ cups each)

1 bunch fresh beets, including greens (about 4 large beets)
1½ teaspoons extra virgin olive oil
2 medium carrots, julienned
1 large onion, halved and sliced into rings
½ medium head (454 g) cabbage, sliced into thin shreds
5 cups (1,185 ml) water
2 reduced sodium vegetable bouillon cubes
2 bay leaves
Juice of ½ lemon
Freshly ground black pepper, to taste
2 tablespoons chopped fresh chives

1. Separate the beets from their greens, reserving the stems and leaves. Trim the beets, remove any rough woody spots, and scrub well. Slice them into matchsticks.

2. Add the olive oil to a large pot over medium heat and add the beets, carrots, and onion. Sauté, stirring occasionally, for 8 minutes.

3. Add the cabbage, water, bouillon, and bay leaves. Stir well, cover, and cook for 20 minutes, until all the vegetables are tender.

4. Meanwhile, coarsely slice the beet leaves and stems. Add to the soup with the lemon juice. Cover and cook for 2 minutes, until leaves are just wilted but still bright green. Add black pepper to taste. Before serving, remove and discard the bay leaves and garnish the soup with the chives.

note: Traditional borscht is often served with a dollop of sour cream. If you'd like to, you can add plant-based sour cream (e.g., Tofutti, Follow Your Heart, or homemade; see page 344) or a dollop of unflavored, unsweetened plant-based yogurt, such as coconut or soy.

PER SERVING: 61 calories, 2 g protein, 12 g carbohdyrate, 1 g fat, 0 g saturated fat, 4 g fiber, 4 g sugar, 169 mg sodium.
STAR NUTRIENTS: folate (11% DV), vitamin A (53% DV), vitamin C (73% DV), vitamin K (147% DV), manganese (13% DV), potassium (13% DV)

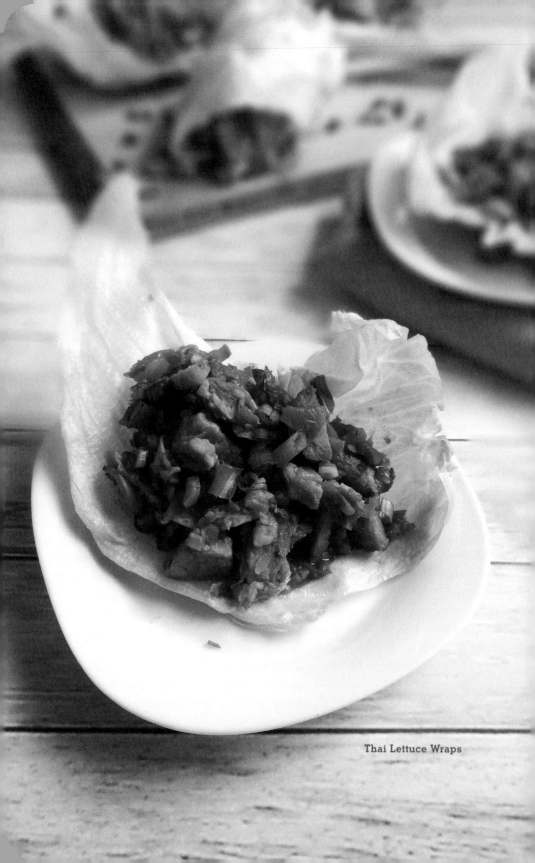

Thai Lettuce Wraps

Foster friendly bacteria.

Black Bean and Corn Chili
Banana-Coconut Brown Rice Pudding
Thai Lettuce Wraps

Your body is composed of a living mass of bacteria—you have about ten times more bacteria in your body than cells. The collection of bacteria—known as the microbiota—in your gut is vital to your health. Your gut bacteria are constantly at war, as "friendly" bacteria duke it out against harmful pathogens and invaders. Scientists are just beginning to uncover the significance of the human gut microbiota; it serves an important role in digestion, but also in immune function and even disease prevention. New studies have even linked gut microbiota to weight—obese people tend to have a different mix of gut bacteria than do thin people. And a new role for gut bacteria is emerging: they appear to unlock phytochemicals to transform them into powerful, bioactive compounds that fight disease (see page 180 for more on phytochemicals).

Your friendly gut bacteria need food to survive and multiply. And what do they eat? Fiber-rich plant foods. That's why Americans, typically eating a highly processed, low-fiber diet, tend to have a dismal profile of gut bacteria. Yet, if you sampled the gut bacteria of a rural villager in Africa, where the diet is heavily plant-based and includes fermented foods (see page 309) rich in live bacteria, you would probably find prolific friendly bacteria.

You have your own personal gut microbiome—your unique community of bacteria. And you can shift its makeup by boosting your diet with lots of fiber-rich, whole plant foods. Only 5 percent of Americans achieve their recommended fiber goal (25 grams per day for women and 38 for men). However, if you eat a plant-powered diet, you can easily exceed it. The best sources of fiber include beans, lentils, peas, and whole grains, such as wheat, oats, rye, and quinoa. Help your friendly bacteria win by feeding them what they want: fiber-rich plant foods.

black bean and corn chili

ACTIVE PREPARATION TIME: **10 minutes** • TOTAL PREPARATION TIME: **1 hour 20 minutes**
(not including soaking time)

One of the best ways to feed your friendly bacteria is to add more fiber-rich legumes to your diet. These foods act as a prebiotic in your gut, encouraging the growth of beneficial bacteria that can improve your digestive function, as well as fuel your immune function. The Southwestern flavors of this black bean chili shine through, making it an excellent cool-weather meal, served with cornbread and a flavorful slaw, such as my Tropical Red Cabbage and Spelt Salad (page 77). Best of all, you can pour all of the ingredients into a slow cooker, set the dial, and come home to a rustic yet satisfying meal at the end of the day.

MAKES 8 SERVINGS
(about 1 cup each)

1 pound (454 g) dried black beans
5 cups (1,183 ml) water, plus more for soaking
1 reduced sodium vegetable broth bouillon cube
2 cups (328 g) frozen sweet corn
1 medium yellow onion, diced
One 6-ounce (170 g) can tomato paste
3 medium garlic cloves, minced
½ tablespoon maple syrup
1 tablespoon barbecue sauce
¼ teaspoon crushed red pepper
1 teaspoon chili powder
¼ teaspoon turmeric
½ teaspoon cumin
Pinch of sea salt, optional

1. Cover the black beans with water and soak overnight.
2. Drain the beans and discard the water. Place the beans in a large pot and add 5 cups of the water, the bouillon cube, corn, onion, tomato paste, garlic, maple syrup, barbecue sauce, crushed red pepper, chili powder, turmeric, cumin, and sea salt, if desired.
3. Cover and bring to a simmer over high heat, then reduce the heat to medium. Cook for about 1 hour 10 minutes, until the chili is thick and the beans are tender, stirring occasionally. You may need to add water to replace moisture lost to evaporation, but the texture should be thick and stewlike.

note: After soaking the beans, you may add all the ingredients to a slow cooker and cook on high for 4 to 5 hours or on low for 8 to 10 hours.

variations: Substitute red beans or pinto beans for the black beans, or use a combination.

PER SERVING: 258 calories, 14 g protein, 51 g carbohydrate, 1 g fat, 0 g saturated fat, 11 g fiber, 6 g sugar, 86 mg sodium
STAR NUTRIENTS: folate (68% DV), niacin (13% DV), riboflavin (10% DV), thiamin (37% DV), vitamin B6 (15% DV), vitamin C (12% DV), iron (20% DV), magnesium (29% DV), potassium (33% DV), zinc (16% DV)

banana-coconut brown rice pudding

ACTIVE PREPARATION TIME: **14 minutes** • TOTAL PREPARATION TIME: **47 minutes**
(not including chilling time)

*Another important group of prebiotics—foods that support the growth
of beneficial bacteria in your gut—are whole grains, rich in a variety of
health-promoting fibers. While you might think your best opportunity to
power up on whole grains is at the breakfast table, it's also possible to
get them at other times—even dessert. My mom made a mean banana
pudding, which was one of my all-time favorite desserts growing up. I
borrowed a trick from her original recipe but featured brown rice.*

MAKES 8 SERVINGS
(about ¾ cup each)

1 cup (196 g) uncooked brown basmati rice
2⅓ cups (552 ml) water
2 cups (474 ml) vanilla coconut milk beverage
1 teaspoon vanilla extract
1 tablespoon cornstarch
½ teaspoon cinnamon
½ teaspoon allspice
2 tablespoons honey or agave nectar
4 small ripe bananas
⅓ cup (47 g) unsweetened shredded coconut or coconut flakes

1. Place the rice and water in a pot, cover, and cook for 30 minutes, stirring occasionally. Drain off any extra water.
2. Meanwhile, in a medium bowl, whisk together the coconut milk, vanilla, and cornstarch with a wire whisk until smooth.
3. When the rice has cooked for 30 minutes, add the coconut milk mixture, cinnamon, allspice, and honey and continue to cook, stirring occasionally, for 15 minutes, until the mixture has thickened into the consistency of porridge and the rice is tender.
4. Mash 2 of the bananas with a fork and stir into cooked rice pudding.
5. Transfer the pudding to a serving dish, cover with plastic wrap (touching the surface of the pudding), and chill for about 2 hours.
6. When ready to serve, slice the remaining 2 bananas into ¼-inch-thick pieces. Top the chilled pudding with the sliced bananas and the coconut.

variation: Substitute another fruit, such as sliced peaches, pineapple chunks, or mango slices, for the bananas, using pureed fruit in step 4, and sliced fruit in step 6.

PER SERVING: 188 calories, 3 g protein, 37 g carbohydrate, 4 g fat, 3 g saturated fat, 3 g fiber, 13 g sugar, 15 mg sodium
STAR NUTRIENTS: vitamin B6 (16% DV), calcium (23% DV), iron (115% DV), magnesium (12% DV), manganese (57% DV), phosphorus (12% DV)

See photo
on page 234

thai lettuce wraps

ACTIVE PREPARATION TIME: **21 minutes** • TOTAL PREPARATION TIME: **21 minutes**

*Thai cuisine offers such bold, fresh flavors in meals that are often based
on plants. In this traditional dish, crisp iceberg lettuce is used to bundle up
a fragrant, spicy mixture of onion, carrot, mushrooms, cabbage, and tempeh. Tempeh, a traditional Indonesian grain and soy food, is an example
of a fermented food that can help boost levels of friendly bacteria in your
gut. These fiber-rich wraps are great warm, but are also good the following
day, chilled and tucked away in your lunch box.*

MAKES 6 SERVINGS
(1 lettuce wrap each)

2 teaspoons peanut oil
½ medium red onion, diced
3 medium garlic cloves, minced
1 teaspoon minced fresh ginger
¼ teaspoon crushed red pepper
4 ounces (113 g) tempeh, diced
1 medium carrot, grated
6 medium button mushrooms, thinly sliced
1 cup (70 g) slivered Chinese (Napa) cabbage
2 tablespoons reduced sodium soy sauce
1 tablespoon honey or agave nectar
Juice of 1 medium lime
3 green onions, white and green parts, chopped
⅓ cup (47 g) chopped peanuts
3 tablespoons chopped mint
3 tablespoons chopped cilantro
1 head iceberg lettuce

1. Heat the peanut oil in a large skillet or wok over medium heat.

2. Add the onion and sauté for 5 minutes.

3. Add the garlic, ginger, crushed red pepper, tempeh, carrot, mushrooms, cabbage, soy sauce, honey, lime juice, green onions, peanuts, mint,
and cilantro. Sauté for an additional 5 to 6 minutes. Do not overcook; the
vegetables should still be crisp and bright.

4. Wash and destem the lettuce and discard any outer leaves that are
wilted or damaged. Peel away 6 whole leaves of lettuce.

5. To create the lettuce wraps, fill each with one sixth of the warm vegetable mixture (generous ½ cup each) using a slotted spoon. Roll up the
leaves burrito fashion and serve warm with the seam side down.

note: Serve warm or chilled the next day. For best results for chilled wraps, store the filling and the lettuce leaves separately and prepare the wraps no more than a few hours before serving.

variation: Substitute tofu, drained and pressed (see page 103), for the tempeh.

PER SERVING: 159 calories, 9 g protein, 15 g carbohydrate, 8.5 g fat, 1.5 g saturated fat, 3 g fiber, 7 g sugar, 208 mg sodium
STAR NUTRIENTS: folate (19% DV), niacin (13% DV), riboflavin (12% DV), thiamin (10% DV), vitamin A (51% DV), vitamin B6 (13% DV), vitamin C (23% DV), vitamin K (57% DV), copper (15% DV), iron (12% DV), magnesium (13% DV), manganese (33% DV), molybdenum (12% DV), phosphorus (16% DV), potassium (10% DV)

California Tofu Scramble

Strengthen your bones with plants.

California Tofu Scramble
Grits Smothered with Mustard Greens
🌱

Keeping your bones strong and healthy is one of the most important things you can do to preserve your health. Diseases such as osteoporosis can make your bones weak and brittle, leading to pain, deformity, and disability as you age. And what you put on your plate day in and day out can have a major impact on the strength of your bones. For plant-powered eaters, it's even more important to pay attention to food choices, because some studies have linked vegetarian (especially) vegan diets with lower bone mineral density.

You've probably already heard that calcium is an important mineral for bone health. If you eat dairy foods, you can meet your calcium needs easily with two to three servings a day. If you don't, you can still get calcium through a plant-based diet, as do many lactose-intolerant populations around the world. Just focus on getting two to three servings of calcium-rich foods every day, such as fortified soy milk, tofu, and orange juice, and green leafy vegetables, almonds, and broccoli.

However, bone nutrition doesn't stop at calcium—vitamin D may be just as important, as it plays a role in bone development. Our ancestors used to get plenty of vitamin D through the sun, as our skin can convert sunlight into this essential vitamin. However, today most people work indoors, cover their bodies in layers of clothing, and live in places that may not get adequate sunlight year-round. Thus, we rely on vitamin D mostly from the fortification of milk, although it is also found in fish. If you eat dairy, you can get your vitamin D through fortified milk, but if not, you can get it in fortified soy milk and orange juice, mushrooms exposed to light (see page 291), and a daily ten-minute dose of sunshine.

If you're concerned about meeting your calcium and vitamin D needs, consider taking a supplement. Other nutrients also support healthy bones, including magnesium and vitamins C and K, readily found in fruits, vegetables, whole grains, nuts, seeds, and legumes. In fact, eating plenty of fruits and vegetables has been linked with bone protection, according to research. It looks like phytochemicals, which have powerful antioxidant properties, may also help boost your bones. So, bone up on a variety of plant-powered foods to keep your bones kicking for life.

california tofu scramble

ACTIVE PREPARATION TIME: **12 minutes** • TOTAL PREPARATION TIME: **14 minutes**

Maximize the power of soy in your diet! Instead of adding animal pro-
teins, like chicken, eggs, or beef, to a dish, just stir in tofu, a traditional
Asian food made from ground soybeans. This tofu scramble, packed with
fresh vegetables, is a perfect plant-powered solution for a late weekend
breakfast or easy meal at the end of a long day. Serve it with whole grain
tortillas, toast, or pita, and a scoop of hummus for an extra protein and
flavor boost.

MAKES 4 SERVINGS
(about 1¼ cups each)

1 teaspoon extra virgin olive oil
½ medium red or white onion, sliced
1 small yellow crookneck squash, sliced
1 small zucchini, sliced
½ medium bell pepper (red, yellow, or green), sliced
1 medium garlic clove, minced
8 ounces (227 g) extra firm tofu, drained and diced small
 (pressed, for best results—see page 103)
½ teaspoon ground cumin
½ teaspoon low-sodium herbal seasoning blend (see page 345)
Pinch of kosher salt, optional
½ medium ripe avocado, peeled and sliced
3 tablespoons fresh cilantro, or 1 teaspoon dried

1. Heat the olive oil in a large skillet over medium heat.

2. Add the onion, squash, zucchini, and bell pepper. Sauté 5 minutes.

3. Add the garlic, tofu, cumin, herbal seasoning, and salt, if desired, and sauté for an additional 5 minutes.

4. Remove from the heat and divide into four servings. Garnish with the sliced avocado and cilantro.

notes: You may substitute one 15-ounce (425 g) can drained beans (e.g., kidney, black, garbanzo, white) for the tofu in step 3.

PER SERVING: 166 calories, 9 g protein, 9 g carbohydrate, 12 g fat, 2 g saturated fat, 5 g fiber, 3 g sugar, 10 mg sodium
STAR NUTRIENTS: folate (12% DV), vitamin B6 (10% DV), vitamin C (57% DV), vitamin K (18% DV), calcium (10% DV), iron (11% DV), magnesium (13% DV), potassium (14% DV)

grits smothered with mustard greens

I am partial to Southern comfort foods thanks to my Arkansas-born mother, who prepared her trademark savory grits and greens on a regular basis. This dish marries these two Southern staples into one easy, nutrient-packed casserole. The bitter greens and caramelized onions partner with the creamy grits beautifully. Add a side of stewed black-eyed peas and you've got a plant-powered match made in heaven. The hefty dose of greens puts this meal off the charts with bone-loving nutrients, such as calcium and vitamin K.

MAKES 8 SERVINGS
(about ½ cup grits with ¾ cup greens)

3 cups (711 ml) water
1 cup (156 g) uncooked corn grits (polenta; see Notes)
1 reduced sodium vegetable bouillon cube
¾ cup (178 ml) unsweetened plain plant-based milk
1 tablespoon extra virgin olive oil
1 large onion, diced
2 medium garlic cloves, minced
Pinch of cayenne pepper (see Notes)
1 teaspoon celery salt
½ teaspoon dry mustard
2 bunches mustard greens (about 20 ounces/567 g total),
   coarsely sliced
1 tablespoons sesame seeds, toasted

1. In a small covered pot over high heat, bring 3 cups of water to a boil. Reduce the heat to medium, add the grits and vegetable bouillon, and stir with a whisk until smooth. Cover the pot and cook for 6 minutes, stirring frequently with a whisk to prevent sticking or lumping. Stir in the plant-based milk, cook for approximately 2 minutes, cover, and remove the pot from the heat. Set aside.

2. While the grits are cooking, heat the olive oil in a very large skillet or sauté pan. Add the onion and sauté for 3 minutes. Add the garlic, cayenne, celery salt, and mustard and sauté for an additional 3 minutes. Pile the sliced mustard greens into the pan and cook for an additional 4 to 5 minutes, until the greens are just wilted, tender, but bright green. Allow the greens to reduce in volume before you start stirring.

3. Pour the hot grits into a large casserole dish or serving dish. Cover with the cooked greens and sprinkle with toasted sesame seeds. Serve immediately.

notes: Look for whole grain grits (such as Bob's Red Mill) made from whole corn, rather than degerminated corn. Some brands of grits call for differing amounts of water; adjust the water as necessary according to package directions.

Increase the amount of cayenne pepper if you like spice.

variations: Try wild greens, such as dandelion greens, lamb's quarters, sorrel, or chickweed, in this recipe. You may require more or less cooking time in step 2, depending on the type of green.

PER SERVING: 128 calories, 4 g protein, 21 g carbohydrate, 3 g fat, 0 g saturated fat, 4 g fiber, 1 g sugar, 223 mg sodium

STAR NUTRIENTS: folate (30% DV), vitamin A (142% DV), vitamin C (156% DV), vitamin K (393% DV), calcium (19% DV), iron (12% DV), manganese (18% DV), potassium (11% DV)

Tempeh Noodle Skillet
with Bok Choy

Make friends with soy.

Tofu Ratatouille
Tempeh Noodle Skillet with Bok Choy

"I heard soy is dangerous." I hear this time and time again. If there's one food that's gotten a bad rap, it's definitely soy. Hundreds of websites malign it, saying that it causes breast cancer, feminizing effects on men, and more. Yet soy, whose history dates back to 1100 BC in China, is one of the most perfect plant foods on the planet—if you had only one food to pack away to survive on a deserted island, soy just might be the best choice. It's not only rich in protein (a "complete" protein, with a good balance of all the essential amino acids), but it's also a good source of twelve essential vitamins and minerals, as well as fiber. Soy contains special phytochemicals called isoflavones, which appear to hold special antioxidant properties that help protect against bone disease, heart disease, and cancer.

These isoflavones, which are phytoestrogens (plant estrogens), are behind much of the confusion on soy. However, most people in Japan eat soy daily in foods such as tofu, miso, and natto (fermented soybean), and they have the highest longevity (and lower prostate and breast cancer rates) among industrialized countries, according to a new analysis.

The American Institute for Cancer Research now says eating one to two daily servings of soy foods is safe (some studies show even up to three servings). I recommend choosing whole soy foods that are minimally processed, such as edamame (the immature soy bean in the pod), cooked soybeans, soy nuts, soy nut butter, tofu, soy milk, tempeh (fermented soy and grain cakes), and miso. You can also find dozens of faux meat products, such as "bacon," "burgers," and "sausages," which are often made of soy protein. While it's fine to store these in the freezer for easy and tasty mealtime solutions, aim to eat most of your soy in its less processed forms.

tofu ratatouille

Tofu—protein-rich, versatile, and easy—is a plant-powered eater's best friend. You can add it to a number of dishes, where it will take on the flavors of the foods with which it is paired. In this traditional vegetable stew from Provence, France, tofu takes on the earthy flavors of sun-ripened vegetables, including eggplant, tomatoes, zucchini, and bell peppers. This rich mélange can hold its own at the center of the plate, especially served with whole grain pasta or steamed farro.

MAKES 8 SERVINGS
(about 1 cup each)

1 tablespoon extra virgin olive oil
1 large onion, diced
2 medium garlic cloves, minced
One 1¼-pound (548 g) eggplant, diced
2 medium zucchinis, diced
1 medium bell pepper (green or yellow), diced
8 ounces (226 g) extra firm tofu, drained and diced (pressed, for
    best results—see page 103)
1 teaspoon dried basil
One 14.5-ounce (411 g) can diced tomatoes, no salt added, with
    liquid
1 cup (257 g) marinara sauce
1 tablespoon capers, rinsed and drained
Freshly ground black pepper to taste
Pinch of sea salt, optional
¼ cup (15 g) chopped fresh parsley

1. Heat the olive oil in a very large sauté pan or Dutch oven over medium heat, add the onion, and cook, stirring frequently, for 7 minutes.
2. Add the garlic, eggplant, zucchini, bell pepper, and tofu to the pan and sauté for an additional 10 minutes.
3. Preheat the oven to 350°F (180°C).
4. Stir the basil, tomatoes, marinara sauce, capers, black pepper, and sea salt, if desired, into the vegetable mixture and cook for an additional 1 to 2 minutes, until bubbling.
5. Transfer the contents to a large casserole dish (about 9 by 13 inches) or leave in the Dutch oven and bake for about 45 minutes, uncovered, until the vegetables are tender. Stir every 15 minutes to distribute the liquid.
6. Remove the dish from the oven, sprinkle with the parsley, and serve immediately.

variations: Omit the tofu for a vegetable side dish. To make Bean Rata-touille with Tofu, rinse and drain one 15-ounce (425 g) can of beans, such as garbanzos or white beans, and add in step 4.

PER SERVING: 115 calories, 6 g protein, 15 g carbohydrate, 4 g fat, .5 g saturated fat, 5 g fiber, 7 g sugar, 294 mg sodium

STAR NUTRIENTS: folate (11% DV), niacin (12% DV), vitamin A (21% DV), vitamin B6 (14% DV), vitamin C (85% DV), vitamin K (51% DV), magnesium (10% DV), manganese (20% DV), potassium (20% DV)

See photo
on page 248

tempeh noodle skillet with bok choy

ACTIVE PREPARATION TIME: **18 minutes** • TOTAL PREPARATION TIME: **18 minutes**

Soy foods have long been an honored tradition in Asia. For example, tempeh harks back about 200 years and still serves as a major source of protein in Indonesia. Here, it adds a flavorful dimension to this stir-fry. Packed with crisp vegetables and Thai spices, this easy one-dish meal showcases the health and flavor benefits of whole soy foods. Plus, you can cook up this healthier take on pad Thai in less time than it would take to pick up takeout.

MAKES 6 SERVINGS
(about 1 cup each)

4 cups (948 ml) water
8 ounces (227 g) uncooked Asian brown rice noodles (e.g., pad Thai noodles)
1 teaspoon peanut oil
1 tablespoon vegetarian Thai chili paste (see Notes)
2 medium garlic cloves
½ teaspoon turmeric
½ teaspoon minced fresh ginger
1 teaspoon coriander
1 teaspoon cumin
½ teaspoon cardamom
¼ teaspoon cloves
½ teaspoon cinnamon
1 cup (237 ml) canned light coconut milk (well mixed before measured)
1 medium bell pepper (yellow or red), sliced
1 cup (70 g) sliced mushrooms
8 ounces (227 g) tempeh, cubed (see Notes)
2 tablespoons reduced sodium soy sauce
¾ cup (72 g) diced green onions, white and green parts
6 ounces (170 g) baby bok choy, trimmed, leaves separated
1 medium lime, quartered
½ cup (30 g) chopped fresh cilantro

1. Bring the water to a boil in a medium pot over high heat. Add rice noodles and cook over medium heat according to package directions (do not overcook). Drain the noodles and rinse. Set aside.

2. Meanwhile, heat the peanut oil over medium heat in a large skillet or wok. Add the chili paste, garlic, turmeric, ginger, coriander, cumin, cardamom, cloves, cinnamon, and 2 tablespoons of the coconut milk. Cook for 1 minute, stirring, to make a paste.

3. Add the bell pepper, mushrooms, and tempeh and sauté for 3 minutes.

4. Stir in the soy sauce and remaining coconut milk and mix well.

5. Add the drained, cooked noodles and ½ cup of the diced green onions and stir well. Place the bok choy leaves on top, cover, and cook for an additional 3 to 4 minutes, until the mixture is heated through and the bok choy leaves are bright green but crisp-tender (to avoid mushiness, do not overcook).

6. Garnish the skillet with the lime quarters, cilantro, and remaining ¼ cup of chopped green onions.

notes: Thai chili paste is a condiment/seasoning available at many supermarkets, as well as Asian stores and online purveyors. Read the ingredients list, since some feature nonvegetarian ingredients.

Tempeh is available in the refrigerated section (with tofu) at many supermarkets, natural food stores, and Asian markets.

variation: You may substitute your favorite Asian noodle for the rice noodles, such as soba, ramen, or udon, and cook according to the package directions in step 1. You may also substitute extra firm tofu (pressed, for best results—see page 103) for the tempeh.

PER SERVING: 270 calories, 11 g protein, 41 g carbohydrate, 8 g fat, 3 g saturated fat, 5 g fiber, 4 g sugar, 380 mg sodium
STAR NUTRIENTS: riboflavin (14% DV), vitamin A (29% DV), vitamin C (75% DV), vitamin K (23% DV), calcium (10% DV), iron (12% DV), magnesium (11% DV), manganese (41% DV), phosphorus (14% DV), potassium (12% DV)

Summer Succotash
with Heirloom Tomatoes

Pay respect to heritage foods.

Cajun Rattlesnake Beans with Corn
Summer Succotash with Heirloom Tomatoes

For nearly every type of plant food, from vegetables to beans, there are hundreds—sometimes thousands—of varieties. These edible plants all started out as wild plants, which bore seeds that gradually traveled around the globe. Eventually, farmers crossbred plants to produce the best crops and saved seeds that were very special—perhaps lovely colored tomatoes, or beans with meaty flesh. As farmers treasured the seeds and handed them down, just as they might pass down their mothers' antique bone china or a handmade quilt, these seeds became known as heirlooms. Their preservation means there are many gorgeous, diverse varieties of edible plants, offering a magnificent range of flavor, texture, and nutrient profiles.

Unfortunately, our vocabulary limits most plant foods to single varieties. You may be familiar only with standard fare, such as small red plum tomatoes, or long-rooted orange Imperator carrots. Yet, heirloom varieties include Cherokee Purple tomatoes and yellow Golden Ball carrots. Quinoa comes in shades of red and black; lentils may be tinged in cheerful yellow, pink, or green; and radishes can be pink and white striped like candy. And, in many cases, the colorful heirloom varieties of plants are even richer in antioxidants than their more familiar cousins.

Over the years, many heritage varieties of plants have been lost, as supermarkets stocked only the most popular varieties. But they are making a comeback. You can find heritage varieties of edible grains, beans, lentils, vegetables, and fruits on today's finest restaurant menus, as well as in farmers markets, some supermarkets, and home gardeners' vegetable seed catalogs. Online purveyors stock heirloom dried corn, grains, beans, and lentils, such as rattlesnake beans and Crimson Popping corn, allowing plant-powered diners flexibility in their daily choices. I have a collection of shelf-stable, nutritious heirlooms in my pantry; I love their colorful names and stories. Along with history, they help provide rich diversity in my diet—as they can in yours. Remember, if you buy it, they will grow it.

cajun rattlesnake beans with corn

ACTIVE PREPARATION TIME: **14 minutes** • TOTAL PREPARATION TIME: **1 hour 45 minutes**
(not including soaking time)

If you're lucky enough to find brown, speckled rattlesnake beans—available in bulk bins in some natural food stores and online—snap them up. They are but just one example of the amazing variety of legumes that have been discovered by farmers, planted, treasured and passed down over the years. The meaty texture of this heirloom bean suits stews and chilies extremely well (although you can substitute another bean if you can't find them). This Cajun-seasoned dish has a spicy bite to match its name.

MAKES 8 SERVINGS
(about 1 cup each)

1½ cups (276 g) dried rattlesnake beans (see Notes)
4 cups (948 ml) water, plus more for soaking
1 teaspoon reduced sodium vegetable broth base
1 cup (237 ml) low-sodium tomato or vegetable juice
1 medium bell pepper (red or green), diced
1 medium tomato, chopped
1 medium onion, chopped
1 cup (101 g) chopped celery
1 cup (128 g) sliced carrots
1 cup (164 g) frozen corn
2 to 3 teaspoons reduced sodium Cajun seasoning, or to taste
   (see page 000)
1 bay leaf
2 medium garlic cloves, minced
1 teaspoon dried thyme

1. Cover the beans with water and soak overnight.
2. Drain the beans and place them in a large pot. Add the water, broth base, tomato juice, bell pepper, tomato, onion, celery, carrots, corn, Cajun seasoning, bay leaf, garlic, and thyme.
3. Stir the contents well, cover, and bring to a simmer over medium heat. Cook for about 1 hour and 30 to 45 minutes, stirring occasionally, until the beans are tender. Taste and adjust the seasonings as desired. Remove the bay leaf before serving.

notes: If rattlesnake beans are not available, substitute kidney beans, red beans, pink beans, cranberry beans, or pinto beans.

You may also cook the chili in a slow cooker on high for 4 to 6 hours or on low for 8 to 10 hours.

PER SERVING: 165 calories, 10 g protein, 32 g carbohydrate, 1 g fat, 0 g saturated fat, 11 g fiber, 5 g sugar, 116 mg sodium
STAR NUTRIENTS: folate (42% DV), riboflavin (11% DV), thiamin (16% DV), vitamin A (68% DV), vitamin B6 (16% DV), vitamin C (98% DV), vitamin K (22% DV), copper (15% DV), iron (18% DV), magnesium (16% DV), manganese (26% DV), phosphorus (15% DV), potassium (22% DV)

See photo
on page 254

summer succotash with heirloom tomatoes

ACTIVE PREPARATION TIME: **17 minutes** • TOTAL PREPARATION TIME: **47 minutes**

I have an ongoing love affair with summer, farm-fresh tomatoes—especially those unusual heirlooms, such as Brandywine and Chocolate Stripe, that offer gorgeous colors and earthy flavors. I feature slabs of heirloom tomatoes in this succotash; however, if needed, you may substitute a more familiar tomato variety, such as Beefsteak and plum, which still provide a rich boost of lycopene. This fresh summer salad showcases two of the "three sisters"—maize (corn), beans, and squash—which formed the backbone of the traditional Native American diet and were traditionally grown together: the corn offered an arbor for the bean vines to climb, and the trailing squash vines grew in their lush canopy.

MAKES: 6 SERVINGS
(about ⅔ cup each)

1 medium ear of corn, shucked (or 1 cup/164 g frozen, thawed corn; see Note)
1½ cups (246 g) frozen lima beans, thawed
1 medium bell pepper (yellow or red), chopped
¼ medium red onion, diced
⅓ cup (23 g) chopped fresh cilantro
1½ tablespoons extra virgin olive oil
2 tablespoons lemon juice
¼ teaspoon freshly ground black pepper
1 teaspoon cumin
1 medium garlic clove, minced
Pinch of sea salt, optional
1 large heirloom (or regular) tomato, thinly sliced

1. Fill a small pot with water and bring to a boil over high heat. Reduce the heat to medium, add the corn, cover, and cook for about 5 minutes, until tender yet firm. Drain, cool, and cut off the corn from the cob.

2. Meanwhile, mix together lima beans, bell pepper, onion, and cilantro in a bowl.

3. In a small dish, whisk together the olive oil, lemon juice, black pepper, cumin, garlic, and sea salt, if desired. Toss into the succotash mixture. Stir in the cooled corn.

4. Line a salad platter with the sliced tomatoes. Pile the succotash over the tomatoes and serve immediately.

note: This is a great recipe for featuring leftover cooked corn on the cob. For even better results, grill the fresh corn for 5 to 10 minutes, until tender and browned, in step 1.

variation: Substitute cooked edamame, fava, garbanzo, or kidney beans for the lima beans.

PER SERVING: 133 calories, 5 g protein, 21 g carbohydrate, 4 g fat, .5 g saturated fat, 4 g fiber, 3 g sugar, 29 mg sodium
STAR NUTRIENTS: folate (10% DV), thiamin (17% DV), vitamin A (11% DV), vitamin B6 (11% DV), vitamin C (130% DV), vitamin K (11% DV), iron (11% DV), magnesium (11% DV), manganese (25% DV), potassium (14% DV)

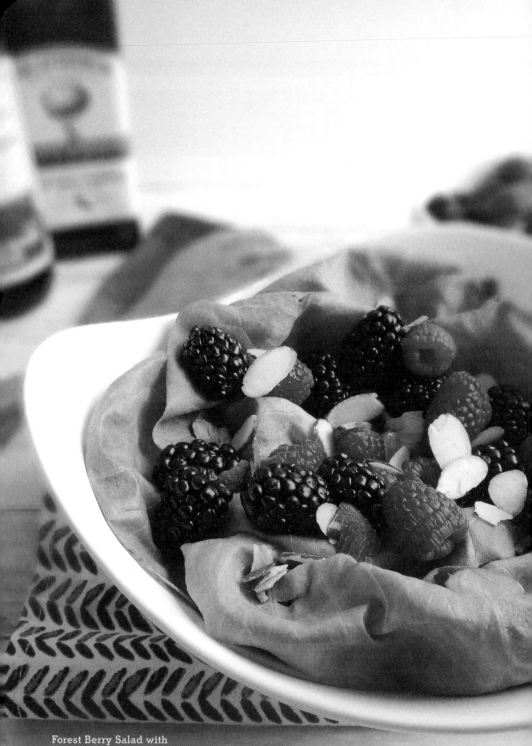

Forest Berry Salad with
Juniper Vinaigrette

Eat mindfully.

Tomato Barley Soup

Forest Berry Salad with Juniper Vinaigrette

❧

Monster muffins, mega cookies, gargantuan meal platters—such are the choices that await you 24/7 everywhere, from bookstores to gas stations. No wonder we're consuming 200 to 500 calories more per day today than we did twenty years ago. You see, science shows that when you are given a portion of food—whether it's a sandwich and fries or a package of snack chips, you tend to eat that portion, no matter its size. Since it takes a while for your brain to get the cues that you're full, you keep eating until the food is gone. And research also shows that you eat more when food is out in the open, such as when you have a bowl of candy on your desk. You also eat more when food is served on bigger plates or even when larger serving spoons are used. And when you eat food in front of the TV or computer, you also can lose track of how much you're eating.

What does all of this mean? It means that you should eat more *mindfully*. Become aware of your eating environment and the eating triggers that can derail you, and learn to enjoy the experience of eating healthfully.

Here are a few suggestions to get you started eating mindfully. First of all, get in touch with your portion sizes. Try to serve up a true portion size for foods, such as one-half cup of hot cereal or cooked pasta, potatoes, or rice; 1 cup of breakfast cereal flakes; 1 ounce of nuts or seeds; or ½ cup of fruit. Now, let your mind fully absorb what that portion size really means and looks like, so that it will be your new normal (this may take eating it several times to sink in). And when you're faced with a multi-serving package of prepared food, such as crackers or trail mix, portion it into single servings rather than polishing off the bag in one sitting.

Second, when you eat, really *enjoy* it. Whenever possible, don't eat your meals while sitting at the computer, watching television, or commuting to the office. Relish the flavors, textures, and bounty of food on your plate, and be *satisfied* with it. You don't have to eat until you feel stuffed to the brim. Consider the Japanese custom called *hara hachi bu*, meaning eating until you feel 80 percent full, which helps Japanese people have much lower rates of obesity than those in many other countries. Mindful eating is essential for finding balance with your weight and health. And be attuned to other signals from your body, too. If, after eating a normal portion of food, you often feel digestive distress, you may be sensitive to one of the ingredients in the meal. Visit a doctor or dietitian to investigate this possibility before removing any foods from your diet.

tomato barley soup

ACTIVE PREPARATION TIME: **12 minutes** • TOTAL PREPARATION TIME: **1 hour 12 minutes**

*Start your meal with a vegetable-based soup, such as this comforting to-
mato barley soup, and you'll be more satisfied at mealtime, says research.
Plus, you'll gain the benefits of the powerful antioxidant lycopene, which
is abundant in tomatoes and has been linked with heart health and cancer
protection. It doesn't get better than this rich soup paired with a toasted
nut butter sandwich!*

MAKES 8 SERVINGS
(about 1 cup each)

5 cups (711 ml) water
2 cups (474 ml) reduced sodium vegetable broth (see page 346)
1 cup (245 g) tomato sauce
¼ cup (66 g) tomato paste
¾ cup (150 g) uncooked barley
1 large garlic clove, minced
1 medium onion, finely diced
1 cup (101 g) diced celery
1 medium carrot, thinly sliced
1 teaspoon thyme
½ teaspoon low-sodium herbal seasoning blend (see page 345)
¼ teaspoon freshly ground black pepper

1. Place the water, broth, tomato sauce, and tomato paste in a large pot
over medium heat and bring to a simmer.
2. Add the barley, garlic, onion, celery, carrot, thyme, herbal seasoning,
and black pepper. Stir well and cover. Reduce the heat to medium-low.
3. Cook for about one hour, until the barley and vegetables are tender. Stir
occasionally and add water as needed to replace moisture lost to evaporation.

note: To make the recipe in a slow cooker, combine all ingredients and cook
on high for 4 to 5 hours or on low for 8 to 10 hours.

variation: For a gluten-free version, substitute buckwheat or brown rice for
the barley.

PER SERVING: 85 calories, 3 g protein, 18 g carbohydrate, .5 g fat, 0 g saturated fat,
4 g fiber, 3 g sugar, 196 mg sodium
STAR NUTRIENTS: vitamin A (34% DV), molybdenum (11% DV), selenium (18% DV)

See photo
on page 260

forest berry salad with juniper vinaigrette

ACTIVE PREPARATION TIME: **6 minutes** • TOTAL PREPARATION TIME: **6 minutes**

Focus on high-nutrient, low-energy foods—namely fruits and vegetables—for a healthy weight and beyond. In fact, if you start your meal with a salad, you can boost your antioxidant intake for the day, as well as increase the satiety value of your meal, which can help you keep your weight on a healthy track. This salad has the extra bonus of berries, which are plant-powered gems packed with special nutrients that may protect your health—brain, heart, and beyond—and provide a naturally sweet, low-calorie, fiber-rich profile perfectly designed to help you feel more satisfied for longer. My salad relies upon wild or cultivated berries of your choosing, and it's flavored with a woodsy juniper vinaigrette that will transport you to the forest where berries originate.

MAKES 4 SERVINGS
(1 generous cup each)

2 teaspoons extra virgin olive oil
1½ teaspoons white balsamic vinegar (see Notes)
½ teaspoon honey or agave nectar
Pinch of sea salt, optional
8 dried juniper berries (see Notes)
3 cups (108 g) packed torn butter lettuce
1½ cups (216 g) assorted fresh berries (e.g., raspberries,
    blueberries, blackberries, salmonberries, sliced strawberries,
    huckleberries)
1½ tablespoons toasted sliced almonds

1. In a medium bowl, whisk together the olive oil, vinegar, honey, and sea salt, if desired, with a fork.
2. Mash the juniper berries using a mortar and pestle (or spoon in a dish) and stir into the bowl.
3. Add the lettuce leaves to the bowl and mix with the vinaigrette using clean hands.
4. Arrange the berries on top of the lettuce. Sprinkle with the almonds just before serving.

notes: Don't substitute regular balsamic vinegar for this recipe, as the color doesn't suit the pale tones of the butter lettuce; however, you can substitute white wine or champagne vinegar.

Dried juniper berries may be found in the spice section of gourmet food stores or online. If you can't find them, substitute a few freshly ground black peppercorns for a different flavor profile.

variations: Substitute chopped romaine, baby spinach, or arugula for the butter lettuce; substitute chopped hazelnuts, walnuts, or pecans for the almonds.

PER SERVING: 67 calories, 2 g protein, 9 g carbohydrate, 4 g fat, 0 g saturated fat, 3 g fiber, 5 g sugar, 1 mg sodium
STAR NUTRIENTS: vitamin A (26% DV), vitamin C (20% DV), vitamin K (13% DV), manganese (12% DV))

Tuscan Kale Salad
with Nectarines
and Brazil Nuts

Learn your foods' pedigree.

Tuscan Kale Salad with Nectarines and Brazil Nuts
Truffled Mashed Gold Potatoes and Celery Root

Start taking an active role in your food supply. Consider: Where did those green peppers in the produce aisle originate? Were the workers who harvested the cocoa beans for your dark chocolate bar paid a decent wage? As you drop items into your shopping cart, you're casting a vote for which foods will flourish in our food system. You aren't an innocent bystander.

Food is a huge part of human life. About 50 percent of the world's land is in farms, and food production accounts for an estimated 20 to 30 percent of global environmental impacts. It also takes up a huge amount of our income— in poor countries, up to 45 percent—so it's worth examining what it is we're paying for so dearly.

It's not the easiest thing to examine. A food's "pedigree" includes issues such as care of the soil, selection of seeds, genetic engineering, use of fertilizers and pesticides, compensation and treatment of farm workers and communities, effects on local wildlife habitats, use and potential contamination of water, humane animal agriculture practices, toxic manure lagoons, animal feed, and the transportation, processing, and distribution of foods. The logistics involved may make your eyes glaze over, or the upsetting facts you uncover may seem overwhelming.

So what's a person to do? Here's a tip that cuts to the heart of most of these issues: eat more minimally processed, organic, locally produced plant foods. I am talking about foods that come the way Mother Nature created them. Think of uncooked barley—essentially the seed of the barley grass dried by the sun and harvested; a bunch of spinach, snipped straight from the soil; a pear, just the way it grew before it was plucked off the tree. The cultivation of whole plant foods, like barley, spinach, and pears, makes a much lower impact on the planet, compared with the production of animal products. Whole plant foods require little to no processing in the form of manufacturing, grinding, mixing with ingredients, packaging, and labeling.

Next, if you can, seek out organic production, which means that the crops are produced without the use of most synthetic pesticides and fertilizers in a method that nurtures the soil and promotes sustainability and biodiversity, and helps protect the farmers who grew your food. And for extra credit, choose seasonal produce from a local grower, which requires fewer fossil fuels to transport to your dinner plate and keeps dollars in your own community.

If you're on a budget, remember that a plant-based diet can be a very cost-effective way to fill your plate. Legumes, grains, and seasonal produce can provide a big nutritional bang for your buck. Don't waste your food dollars on organic junk food, such as chips and crackers. Save them for fruits, vegetables, grains, and legumes—especially those that have no protective coating against pesticide application, such as grapes, lettuce, and peppers. Look for organic produce bargains at your local farmers market and CSA (see page 99). Over time, this eating style can yield vast rewards.

tuscan kale salad with nectarines and brazil nuts

See photo
on page 266

ACTIVE PREPARATION TIME: 10 minutes • TOTAL PREPARATION TIME: 10 minutes

While kale is trendy these days, it was even more popular in the Middle Ages when it was one of the most widely eaten vegetables. This leafy green is actually in the cabbage family, meaning it has anti-cancer compounds, as well as a host of vitamins and minerals. Don't be afraid to experiment with a variety of kales, from Russian to curly leaf. For example, this salad calls upon the deep purple-green of lacinato (Tuscan) kale to form a pretty landscape for the bright, fresh nectarines. And you might want to prioritize organic when you select these ingredients—both kale and nectarines show up on the top twenty list for pesticide residues, according to the Environmental Working Group.

MAKES 10 SERVINGS
(about 1¼ cups each)

1 large bunch Tuscan (lacinato) kale (about 10 ounces/283 g, or
    8 cups loosely packed), washed, dried, and sliced (see Note)
1½ tablespoons extra virgin olive oil
1 tablespoon lemon juice
1 teaspoon whole grain mustard
¼ teaspoon freshly ground black pepper
Pinch of sea salt, optional
2 tablespoons finely diced shallots
3 medium fresh nectarines, sliced, with skins
⅓ cup (44 g) coarsely chopped Brazil nuts

1. Place the kale in a large salad bowl.
2. In a small dish, whisk together olive oil, lemon juice, mustard, black pepper, and a pinch of sea salt, if desired. Stir in the shallots.
3. Pour the dressing over the kale and massage it in with your hands for about 30 seconds, until well distributed.
4. Toss in the nectarines. Sprinkle with the Brazil nuts. Serve immediately.

note: Bagged, prewashed, chopped kale works well in this recipe.

PER SERVING: 80 calories, 2 g protein, 8 g carbohydrate, 5 g fat, 1 g saturated fat, 2 g fiber, 4 g sugar, 77 mg sodium
STAR NUTRIENTS: vitamin A (59% DV), vitamin C (62% DV), vitamin K (254% DV), copper (28% DV), manganese (14% DV), selenium (109% DV)

truffled mashed gold potatoes and celery root

ACTIVE PREPARATION TIME: **11 minutes** • TOTAL PREPARATION TIME: **35 minutes**

Make the most of local, organic foods, especially when it comes to root vegetables, including golden potatoes and celery root, which lends a lighter, herbal taste to classic mashed potatoes. All it takes is a drizzle of precious truffle oil—made from olive oil infused with the flavors of truffles—to amp up the savory factor in this simple side dish. It's a rare and expensive treat to sample truffles, the underground fungi called "the diamonds of the kitchen." However, truffle oil, usually flavored with truffle essence instead of real truffles, can provide that rich, aromatic flavor for a fraction of the price. Look for truffle oil in gourmet food stores, and knobby celery roots in farmers markets or natural food stores.

MAKES 8 SERVINGS
(about ¾ cup each)

6 medium gold potatoes (680 g total), such as Yukon, with peels, halved
2 small celery roots (510 g total), peeled and halved
1½ tablespoons truffle oil
1 to 1¼ cups (237 to 296 ml) unsweetened plain plant-based milk
¼ teaspoon white pepper
Pinch of sea salt, optional
⅓ cup (32 g) sliced green onions, green parts

1. Place the potato and celery root halves in a large pot and cover with water. Cover and bring to a boil over medium-high heat. Reduce the heat to medium and cook for about 20 minutes, until the vegetables are tender when pierced with a fork.
2. Drain the vegetables and add 1 tablespoon of the truffle oil, 1 cup of the plant-based milk, and the white pepper. Mash with a potato masher or electric mixer until thick, with some lumps. Add additional plant-based milk if needed to create a creamy texture. Taste and add salt, if desired.
3. Pile the mashed vegetables onto a serving plate or casserole dish. Drizzle with the remaining ½ tablespoon truffle oil and garnish with the green onions. Serve immediately.

variations: Substitute another flavored olive oil, such as basil, garlic, chili, or lemon, for the truffle oil to create a new flavor profile.

PER SERVING: 131 calories, 4 g protein, 22 g carbohydrate, 4 g fat, .5 g saturated fat, 4 g fiber, 2 g sugar, 74 mg sodium
STAR NUTRIENTS: vitamin B6 (18% DV), vitamin C (37% DV), vitamin K (38% DV), manganese (12% DV), phosphorus (12% DV), potassium (16% DV)

Strawberry
Soy Lassi

Sport a plant-based milk mustache.

Baked Potato and Leek Soup
Strawberry Soy Lassi

❦

Plant-based milk is so much more than a substitute for dairy. Soy milk first hit the scene in China in AD 82, and today, you can find milks made of nuts, grains, seeds, and legumes: soy, rice, almonds, hazelnuts, oats, hemp, sunflower, coconut, and flax milk. There's a lot to love about these plant-based alternatives nutritionally—they may contain good sources of protein, calcium, and vitamin D—and they work just like dairy milk in your morning cereal or coffee, smoothies, blended soups, and baking.

By swapping a plant-based milk alternative for dairy milk every day, you can power up your diet and reduce your environmental impact—it takes 77 percent less water to make one half-gallon of plant-based milk than it does to make the same amount of dairy milk. Just remember to be selective, as some varieties may have unwanted ingredients, such as sweeteners and flavorings, and many (except soy and protein-fortified plant-based milks) are low in protein. Choose a brand made with organic ingredients and no added sweeteners, and that provides at least 30% DV for calcium and vitamin D and at least 6 grams of protein per serving. You could even make your own at home by soaking, cooking, and grinding grains, legumes, or nuts before blending them with water and straining the liquid.

Many plant-based milks are shelf-stable, so you can stock up on a variety for different uses. The nutritional profile of organic, unsweetened, plain soy milk makes it a great choice for everyday use, but creamy, snow-white coconut milk performs wonderfully in baked goods and creamy desserts. Discover your own favorite traditions for plant-based milk today.

baked potato and leek soup

ACTIVE PREPARATION TIME: **15 minutes** • TOTAL PREPARATION TIME: **1 hour 20 minutes**

This quintessential comfort food soup—reminiscent of a freshly baked potato straight from the oven—now receives the plant-powered treatment. It's so rich and creamy, you won't believe that it's made with plant-based milk and cheese! It's so satisfying that it's almost a meal on its own, but I suggest you round out your meal with a complementary, protein-rich salad, such as Spicy Black-Eyed Pea Salad (page 162). This soup is great the next day, too.

MAKES 6 SERVINGS
(about 1¼ cups each)

4 small baking potatoes, such as russet, with peels (680 g total; see Notes)
2 teaspoons extra virgin olive oil
1 medium leek (white and green parts), trimmed and sliced
¾ cup (178 ml) plus 1 tablespoon water
3 cups (711 ml) unsweetened plain plant-based milk
3 tablespoons all purpose flour
Freshly ground black pepper
½ teaspoon thyme
½ teaspoon low-sodium herbal seasoning blend (see page 345)
Pinch of sea salt, optional
⅓ cup (37 g) shredded plant-based cheddar cheese
2 tablespoons chopped fresh chives

1. Preheat the oven to 350°F (180°C).

2. Place the potatoes in a small baking dish and pierce with a fork. Drizzle 1 teaspoon of the olive oil over the potatoes and bake for about 1 hour and 10 minutes, until tender when pressed.

3. After about 40 minutes, place the leeks in another small baking dish. Drizzle with the remaining 1 teaspoon of olive oil and 1 tablespoon of water. Bake (with the potatoes) for about 30 minutes, until tender and browned.

4. About 10 minutes before removing the vegetables, add the plant-based milk to a medium pot. Stir in the flour with a whisk and cook, stirring frequently, over medium-high heat, until smooth and bubbly, 4 to 5 minutes. Add the ¾ cup of water and the black pepper, thyme, and herbal seasoning. Cook, stirring, for an additional 2 to 3 minutes, until the soup is thick and bubbly. Turn off the heat and cover.

5. When the vegetables are tender, remove from the oven. Let the potatoes cool enough to handle, then dice them, without peeling. Stir the potatoes and leeks into the soup. Taste and add sea salt, if desired.

6. To serve, fill six soup bowls with about 1¼ cups of soup, and top each with 1 tablespoon plant-based cheese and 1 teaspoon chives. Serve immediately.

notes: If you cannot find small baking potatoes, use 2 large baking potatoes and cook until tender (cooking time may increase slightly). This is an excellent recipe for using up leftover baked potatoes (use in step 5).

For a speedier version of this recipe, microwave the potatoes in step 2 for 8 to 12 minutes, until tender. Refrigerate any leftovers and reheat on the stovetop or in the microwave, garnishing with cheese and chives when hot.

variation: To make this dish gluten-free, substitute 2 tablespoons cornstarch for the flour and check that all other ingredients are gluten-free.

PER SERVING: 205 calories, 9 g protein, 26 g carbohydrate, 7 g fat, 1 g saturated fat, 4 g fiber, 3 g sugar, 106 mg sodium.
STAR NUTRIENTS: folate (17% DV), niacin (10% DV), riboflavin (20% DV), thiamin (21% DV), vitamin A (22% DV), vitamin B6 (23% DV), vitamin C (25% DV), vitamin K (26% DV), calcium (28% DV), iron (15% DV), magnesium (15% DV), potassium (21% DV)

See photo
on page 272

strawberry soy lassi

ACTIVE PREPARATION TIME: **4 minutes** • TOTAL PREPARATION TIME: **4 minutes**

In the hot, humid climate of parts of India, a lassi—a yogurt-based, fruity, spicy drink—is a welcome relief. My plant-powered version relies on soy yogurt and soy milk for a creamy texture without skimping on nutrition. Soy milk and yogurt, richest in protein of all of the plant-based milk products, offer a great nutritional profile to this beverage, making it a great snack or complement to an Indian-inspired meal.

MAKES 1 SERVING
(about 1¼ cups)

½ cup (83 g) sliced fresh strawberries (see Note)
½ cup (113 g) strawberry-flavored cultured soy yogurt
¼ cup (59 ml) unsweetened plain soy milk
¼ teaspoon cardamom
½ teaspoon vanilla extract
3 ice cubes

1. Place all ingredients in a blender and process for about 10 seconds, until smooth.
2. Serve immediately.

note: You may use frozen, thawed strawberries.

variation: Substitute blueberries or peaches for the strawberries and use blueberry- or peach-flavored soy yogurt. You may also substitute another plant-based milk or yogurt for soy.

PER SERVING: 160 calories, 5 g protein, 29 g carbohydrate, 2.5 g fat, 0 g saturated fat, 3 g fiber, 19 g sugar, 40 mg sodium
STAR NUTRIENTS: vitamin C (115% DV), calcium (30% DV), manganese (22% DV)

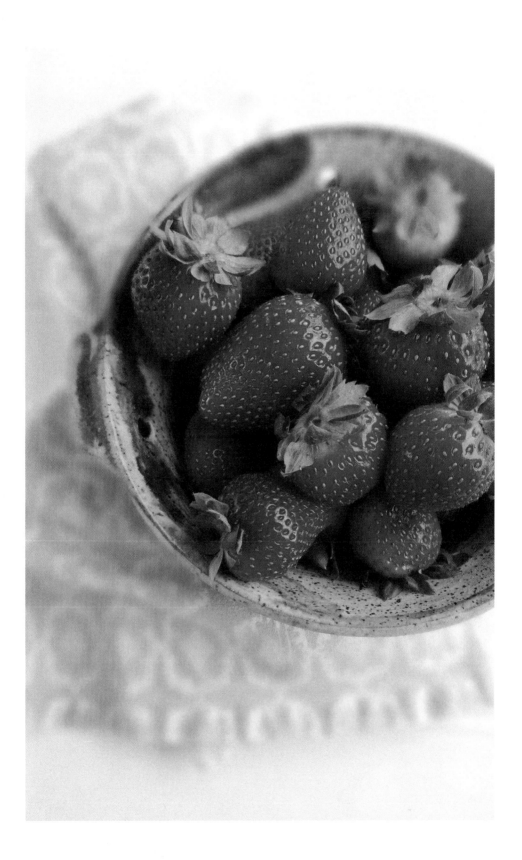

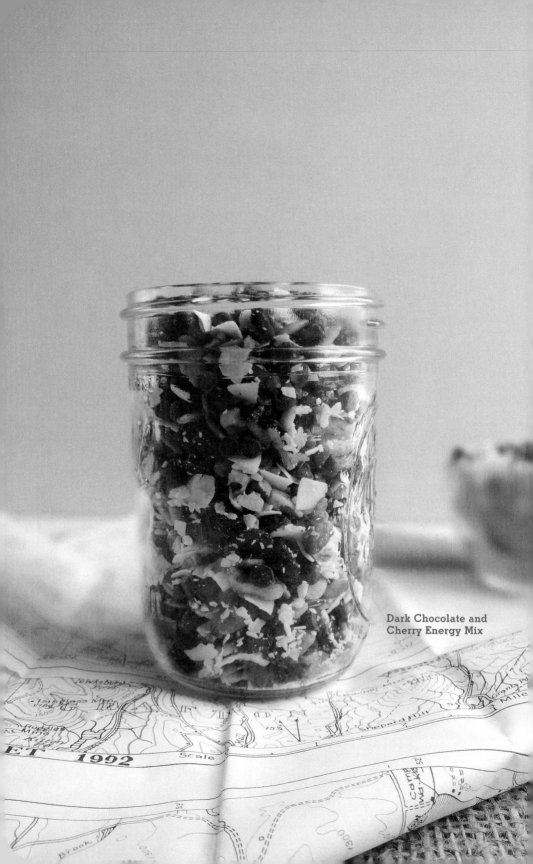

Dark Chocolate and
Cherry Energy Mix

Get a daily plant-powered omega-3 boost.

Banana-Walnut-Flax Bread
Crunchy Farro-Hemp Breakfast Bowl with Fresh Berries
Dark Chocolate and Cherry Energy Mix

What's so special about flax, chia, and walnuts? They contain omega-3 fatty acids—the superstars of the healthy fats world. These unsaturated fats are vital for your health; they reduce inflammation that can lead to disease, and defend you against heart disease and strokes. There's even evidence that omega-3s help protect the brain by fighting Alzheimer's disease and depression.

There are two types of omega-3s: long-chain (docosahexaenoic acid, or DHA, and eicosapentaenoic acid, or EPA) and short-chain (alpha-linolenic acid, or ALA). Much of the evidence on omega-3 benefits is attributed to DHA and EPA, found in seafood. ALA, found in plant food sources, like walnuts and flax, can be converted modestly into DHA and EPA. And ALA has its own anti-inflammatory and heart health benefits, too.

Omega-3s are so key to optimal health that you should fit them into your diet every day. Vegetarians and vegans can get DHA and EPA from supplements made of marine algae—which is where fish get their omega-3s in the first place. If you do eat seafood, aim for at least two servings a week for an average of 250 milligrams of DHA and EPA combined per day.

A daily dose of about 800 to 1,100 milligrams of ALA is also recommended. You can easily achieve this amount by eating plants such as flax, chia, and hemp seeds; walnuts; and soy foods. I start out most days with a bowl of whole grain porridge, such as oats, teff, or quinoa, and I mix in flax, chia, hemp, or walnuts. If you try this, too, along with seasonal fruit and a splash of soy milk, you'll enjoy a delicious, satisfying meal, plus get your daily omega-3 boost first thing in the morning.

banana-walnut-flax bread

ACTIVE PREPARATION TIME: **12 minutes** • TOTAL PREPARATION TIME: **1 hour 12 minutes**

You'll be surprised to discover that this light, moist bread contains no eggs and is sweetened naturally with ripe bananas and a touch of agave. As an added bonus, it's rich in heart-healthy fats: olive oil for a dose of monounsaturated fats, and chia seeds, flaxseeds, and walnuts for a rush of omega-3 fatty acids (each slice packs 930 milligrams!). Slice this whole-some banana bread to accompany a salad or soup for lunch, enjoy it at your coffee or tea break, or serve it as a wholesome dessert.

MAKES 1 LOAF
(12 servings, 1 slice each)

Nonstick cooking spray
3 very ripe medium bananas, mashed (354 g total)
⅓ cup (73 g) extra virgin olive oil
⅓ cup (113 g) honey or agave nectar
2 tablespoons chia seeds (see Notes on page 139)
2 tablespoons ground flaxseeds
1 teaspoon baking soda
1½ cups (180 g) whole wheat flour (see Note)
⅓ cup (39 g) finely chopped walnuts
½ teaspoon cinnamon
¼ teaspoon allspice
¼ teaspoon cardamom

1. Preheat the oven to 350°F (180°C). Spray a 9 by 5-inch loaf pan with nonstick cooking spray.
2. In a medium mixing bowl, mix the bananas, olive oil, honey, chia seeds, and flaxseeds together with an electric mixer or whisk vigorously for 2 minutes, until fluffy.
3. Add the baking soda, flour, walnuts, cinnamon, allspice, and cardamom and stir only until well combined.
4. Pour the batter into the prepared pan and bake for about 1 hour, until the bread is golden brown and a fork inserted into the center comes out clean.
5. Let the bread cool for about 10 minutes, then remove from the pan. Cool slightly before slicing.

note: For a more tender bread, use white whole wheat flour or whole wheat pastry flour.

variations: Substitute hemp seeds for the flaxseeds, and pecans, almonds, or hazelnuts for the walnuts. To make this recipe gluten-free, substitute 1¼ cups of a gluten-free flour blend (such as Bob's Red Mill or King Arthur Flour) for the whole wheat flour. Confirm that all other ingredients are gluten-free.

PER SERVING: 197 calories, 3 g protein, 27 g carbohydrate, 10 g fat, 1 g saturated fat, 4 g fiber, 12 g sugar, 107 mg sodium
STAR NUTRIENTS: vitamin B6 (10% DV), vitamin C (11% DV), magnesium (11% DV), manganese (46% DV), selenium (16% DV)

crunchy farro-hemp breakfast bowl with fresh berries

ACTIVE PREPARATION TIME: **5 minutes** • TOTAL PREPARATION TIME: **37 minutes**

Breakfast is a great way to get your omega-3s. Simply stir omega-rich nuts and seeds, such as hemp, into your whole grain cereal, and you're good to go! I love to turn to ancient grains for simple breakfast solutions. When combined with fruit, nuts, and seeds, this cereal bowl, based on the ancient Roman grain farro, packs fiber, vitamins, minerals, protein, and low-glycemic carbs into your morning, which will leave you satisfied until lunchtime.

MAKES 4 SERVINGS
(about ¾ cup of cereal and ½ cup of berries each)

1 cup (200 g) uncooked farro
3 cups (711 ml) water
1 teaspoon pure vanilla extract
½ teaspoon cinnamon
2 tablespoons hemp seeds
⅓ cup (36 g) chopped pecans
2 cups (288 g) fresh berries (sliced strawberries, blueberries, raspberries, and/or blackberries; see Notes)
Plant-based milk, optional

1. Place the farro in a small pot with the water. Cook, covered, over medium heat for 25 minutes, until tender.
2. Stir in the vanilla, cinnamon, hemp seeds, and pecans, and cook for an additional 5 minutes
3. Divide the cereal into four servings.
4. Top each serving with ½ cup of berries.
5. Serve with plant-based milk, if desired.

notes: Substitute frozen berries for the fresh berries if it is not berry season near you.

You may make one batch and store it in an airtight container in the refrigerator to reheat individually during the week; in this case, reserve the pecans and fruit to add after reheating.

This recipe provides an omega-3 boost of 600 milligrams.

variation: Substitute quinoa or brown rice for the farro in step 1, and add required amount of water and cook according to the package directions.

PER SERVING: 288 calories, 10 g protein, 43 g carbohydrate, 8 g fat, .5 g saturated fat, 7 g fiber, 5 g sugar, 37 mg sodium

STAR NUTRIENTS: riboflavin (12% DV), thiamin (13% DV), vitamin B6 (10% DV), vitamin C (72% DV), iron (17% DV), magnesium (26% DV), manganese (36% DV), phosphorus (24% DV), potassium (11% DV), zinc (12% DV)

See photo
on page 278

dark chocolate and cherry energy mix

ACTIVE PREPARATION TIME: **4 minutes** • TOTAL PREPARATION TIME: **4 minutes**

Make your own energy mix, starring whole nuts, dried fruits, seeds, and dark chocolate pieces. Pack it as a snack, sprinkle it over fruit or plant-based yogurt, or stir it into breakfast cereal. The walnuts and chia seeds give this trail mix a rush of omega-3s—providing almost 1,200 milligrams per serving. And boosting omega-3s is a good thing, as these healthy fats have been linked with reducing inflammation and protecting against heart disease. Keep this mix on hand as a great contribution to any day.

MAKES 12 SERVINGS
(about ½ cup each)

....

½ cup (58 g) walnuts halves
½ cup (55 g) pecans halves
1 cup (227 g) shelled pumpkin seeds
1 cup (93 g) unsweetened dried coconut
1 cup (120 g) unsweetened dried blueberries
1 cup (120 g) unsweetened dried cherries
1 cup (170 g) dairy-free dark chocolate chips
¼ cup (52 g) chia seeds

1. Mix all the ingredients together in a large airtight container and store for up to 3 weeks in a cool, dark place. You may also freeze it for up to 6 months.

variations: Substitute peanuts, almonds, hazelnuts, and/or macadamia nuts for the pecans; sunflower seeds for the pumpkin seeds; and/or raisins for the blueberries.

PER SERVING: 312 calories, 3 g protein, 35 g carbohydrate, 19 g fat, 8.5 g saturated fat, 8 g fiber, 15 g sugar, 14 mg sodium
STAR NUTRIENTS: copper (13% DV), magnesium (11% DV), manganese (34% DV)

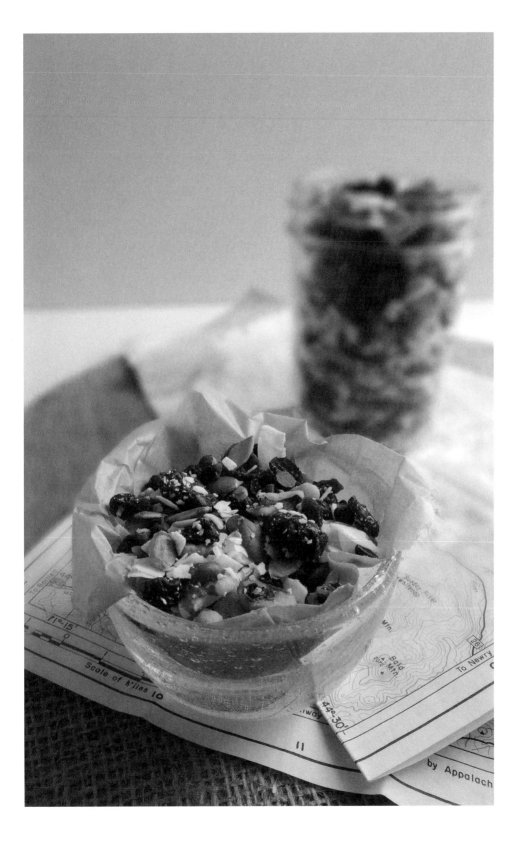

Tropical Green
Smoothie

Become a smoothie operator.

Fruit and Almond Breakfast Shake
Tropical Green Smoothie

Smoothies are a great way to boost your diet with nutrients you may be falling short on, such as protein and calcium. Plus, people of all ages—from kids to seniors—love a delicious, fruit-filled smoothie. Unlike many juicers, which force you to discard nutritious pulp, peels, and fiber, smoothies grind up everything into one thick, easy-to-drink beverage. A well-designed smoothie can serve as a quick meal replacement, as well as a perfect dessert or snack, especially pre- or post-workout. You can design your own smoothie by asking yourself:

- What foods am I falling short on (e.g., fruits, veggies, dairy alternatives, green leafies)?
- What nutrients am I falling short on (e.g., calcium, vitamin D, omega-3 fatty acids, protein)?
- What are my favorite flavors?

Now, create your own unique smoothie that will provide important servings of foods and nutrients perfect for you. Fill your blender with the following, and then whizz away.

- Start with fruit, such as bananas, frozen berries, or mango.
- Toss in some veggies, such as kale, spinach, avocado, or cucumbers. It may take time to get used to the taste of veggies in your smoothie, so start with a small amount and increase as you become more accustomed.
- Select a plant-based milk that suits your needs and taste. Keep in mind that soy milk and fortified almond milk are currently the only plant-based milks that provide a good source of protein.
- Boost the nutrition and flavor:
    * Omega-3: flax, hemp, or chia seeds or walnuts
    * Protein: hemp powder, nuts or nut butter, or peanut butter
    * Flavor: dark chocolate, vanilla, mint leaves, or coconut extract

fruit and almond breakfast shake

ACTIVE PREPARATION TIME: **6 minutes** • TOTAL PREPARATION TIME: **6 minutes**

A quick, wholesome breakfast on the run is minutes away, with the help of a blender. My breakfast shake has all of the elements of a plant-powered meal: fruits, whole grains, nuts, and seeds all wrapped (or whizzed) up in a glass. You can get a day's worth of vitamin C and another 10 percent or more of ten other essential nutrients, including calcium and iron.

MAKES 2 SERVINGS
(about 1½ cups each)

1 medium orange, peeled and sectioned (see Note)
1 cup (155 g) frozen berries (strawberries, raspberries, blackberries, and/or blueberries)
½ cup (119 ml) orange juice
1 cup (237 ml) unsweetened plain almond milk
2 tablespoons almond butter
2 tablespoons flaxseeds
½ cup (78 g) uncooked old-fashioned oats
1 teaspoon pure vanilla extract

1. Combine all the ingredients in a blender and process until smooth (about 2 minutes). Serve immediately.

note: You may substitute 1 cup (189 g) canned, drained mandarin orange for the fresh orange. For a higher-protein shake, use protein-fortified almond milk.

variations: You may add ½ cup greens, such as kale, arugula, or spinach. You may substitute peaches, mangoes, or bananas for the berries.

> **PER SERVING:** 338 calories, 8 g protein, 46 g carbohydrate, 16 g fat, 1 g saturated fat, 9 g fiber, 21 g sugar, 80 mg sodium
> **STAR NUTRIENTS:** folate (14% DV), riboflavin (12% DV), thiamin (13% DV), vitamin C (125% DV), vitamin E (26% DV), calcium (20% DV), iron (13% DV), magnesium (25% DV), manganese (20% DV), phosphorus (20% DV), potassium (16% DV)

tropical green smoothie

See photo
on page 286

*This ice-cool smoothie is green as spring grass, but the tropical notes
of mango, coconut, and pineapple mellow out any potential bitterness.
Packed with heart-healthy nutrients—beta-carotene, vitamin C, and fiber—
it's a great breakfast beverage on the run, snack, or meal accompaniment.*

MAKES 2 SERVINGS
(1¼ cups each)

½ cup (10 g) packed arugula leaves
½ cup (123 g) frozen pineapple chunks
½ cup (83 g) frozen mango chunks
½ large fresh or frozen banana
¼ cup (59 ml) orange juice
1 cup (237 ml) unsweetened plain coconut milk beverage
1 tablespoon hemp seeds
½ teaspoon pure coconut extract or flavoring (see Note)

1. Combine all the ingredients in a blender and process for about 1 to 2
minutes, until smooth. Pour into two glasses and serve immediately.

note: For the best flavor, look for pure coconut extract or flavoring, made
from real coconuts and available in gourmet food stores and online, instead
of imitation coconut extract, which is made from artificial flavorings.

variations: You may substitute fresh or frozen baby spinach for the arugula, and soy or almond milk for the coconut milk.

PER SERVING: 160 calories, 7 g protein, 26 g carbohydrate, 4 g fat, .5 g saturated fat,
3 g fiber, 18 g sugar, 50 mg sodium
STAR NUTRIENTS: folate (12% DV), riboflavin (19% DV), thiamin (18% DV), vitamin A (21% DV),
vitamin B6 (15% DV), vitamin C (94% DV), vitamin K (80% DV), calcium (17% DV), copper
(14% DV), iron (15% DV), magnesium (11% DV), manganese (34% DV), potassium (13% DV)

Portobello Mushroom
and Spinach Pie

Discover the magic of mushrooms.

Savory Shiitake and White Bean Bake
Broccoli-Mushroom Gratin
Portobello Mushroom and Spinach Pie

Mushrooms are not truly plants, but nor are they animal—they belong in the realm of fungi, carrying spores to continue the life of a fungal organism. The planet is packed with thousands of different kinds of mushrooms, most of them still waiting in dark jungles and forests to be discovered by scientists. (Mushroom hunting in the wild has been practiced for centuries, but you must be experienced to avoid picking and eating inedible mushrooms that contain toxic compounds.)

Besides their botanical classification, what's so special about the mysterious mushroom? For starters, they have been used as traditional medicine for centuries and are in fact the source of some of today's most successful drugs: statins and penicillin, for example. These unusual organisms contain all sorts of nutrients, such as fibers, vitamins, and trace elements—but they also contain totally unique bacteria, yeasts, and molds. Even more intriguing is that mushrooms can capture sunlight and turn it into vitamin D, just like we can, so mushrooms that have been exposed to sunlight during their cultivation can be a good source of this elusive vitamin. You can find these at the store, labeled "UV-treated mushrooms." Today, doctors in parts of Asia use mushrooms as a cancer treatment, and mushrooms are being studied for their cancer-fighting effects elsewhere as well, including in the United States.

But beyond all of the nutrients and health-protective qualities tucked away in mushrooms, there's yet another reason to love them. They offer a "meaty," savory quality, rare in the plant world, called umami—one of the five basic taste senses, which also include sweet, sour, salty, and bitter. Mushrooms' umami, along with their "meaty" texture, can give plant-powered foods a rich appeal. For health and pleasure, include a variety of mushrooms—brown, white, oyster, shiitake, chanterelle, enoki, portobello, and more—in your meal plan. Enjoy them sautéed in breakfast scrambles, stir-fried with brown rice, marinated and grilled whole, sliced onto salads, simmered in soups, and folded into casseroles.

savory shiitake and white bean bake

ACTIVE PREPARATION TIME: **12 minutes** • TOTAL PREPARATION TIME: **1 hour 20 minutes**
(not including soaking time)

The savory, umami flavors of shiitake and white beans meld into this nutritious, easy bean bake. Mushrooms—rich in meaty texture and health-protective nutrients—are a perfect match for plant-powered eating. Just serve these beans with a grain dish, such as Stir-Fried Barley with Sea Vegetables and Peanuts (page 132) and a salad, like Tuscan Kale Salad with Nectarines and Brazil Nuts (page 269).

MAKES 6 SERVINGS
(1 scant cup each)

2 cups (430 g) dried white beans
4¼ cups (1,185 ml) water, plus more for soaking
1 teaspoon reduced sodium vegetable broth base
1 tablespoon tomato paste
½ tablespoon extra virgin olive oil
1 medium leek, white part, trimmed and sliced
3.5 ounces (99 g or about 1½ cups) sliced shiitake mushrooms
   (see Note)
2 medium garlic cloves, minced
1 teaspoon dried thyme
¼ teaspoon black pepper
1 teaspoon reduced sodium soy sauce
1 bay leaf

1. Cover the white beans with water and soak overnight. Drain and add beans to a large pot.
2. Add the water, broth base, and tomato paste to the pot, cover, and bring to a boil over high heat. Reduce the heat to medium and simmer for about 5 minutes.
3. Meanwhile, heat the olive oil in a skillet over medium heat, add the leek, and sauté for 2 minutes. Add the mushrooms, garlic, thyme, black pepper, and soy sauce and continue to sauté for 3 minutes, until the mixture is golden.
4. Add the mushroom mixture and bay leaf to the beans. Stir well, cover, and continue simmering over medium heat for about 1 hour, until the beans are tender and the mixture is thick. Add water as needed to replace moisture lost to evaporation.
5. About 5 minutes before the beans are done, preheat the oven to 375°F (190°C).

6. Place the beans in a casserole dish and bake, uncovered, for about 20 minutes, until bubbly and golden. Remove the bay leaf before serving.

note: You may substitute ¾ cup dried shiitake mushrooms for fresh; adding them in step 2 instead of step 3.

variation: Substitute another bean variety, such as pink beans, small kidney beans, or heirloom beans for the white beans. You may also substitute a different type of mushroom for the shiitake, such as oyster, cremini, or white button.

PER SERVING: 245 calories, 16 g protein, 44 g carbohydrate, 2 g fat, 0 g saturated fat, 11 g fiber, 3 g sugar, 60 mg sodium
STAR NUTRIENTS: folate (65% DV), thiamin (20% DV), vitamin B6 (14% DV), vitamin K (18% DV), calcium (17% DV), copper (38% DV), iron (46% DV), magnesium (33% DV), manganese (73% DV), potassium (36% DV), selenium (15% DV), zinc (18% DV)

---

broccoli-mushroom gratin

ACTIVE PREPARATION TIME: 15 minutes • TOTAL PREPARATION TIME: 50 minutes

This classic American side gets a plant-powered remake, thanks to a few pantry staples, fresh broccoli, and meaty, savory mushrooms. You won't believe how creamy and flavorful this dairy-free version is! Plus, it's easy to whip up on the spur of the moment. Let it star as the perfect companion for baked potatoes at dinner, and try it heated up for lunch the next day.

MAKES 6 SERVINGS
(1 cup each)

1½ teaspoons extra virgin olive oil
½ medium onion, halved and sliced into thin rings
1 medium garlic clove, minced
¼ teaspoon dry mustard
1 teaspoon thyme
½ teaspoon low-sodium herbal seasoning blend (see page 345)
¼ teaspoon black pepper, freshly ground
Pinch of kosher salt, optional
1 small bunch broccoli (about 3¾ cups, 12 ounces, or 340 g),
    broken into broccoli florets (see Notes)
2 cups (140 g) sliced white mushrooms (see Notes)
1 tablespoon water
2 tablespoons all-purpose flour
1½ cups (356 ml) unsweetened plain plant-based milk (for best
    results, use coconut milk beverage)
¼ cup (28 g) plant-based cheese, optional
2 tablespoons whole grain bread crumbs (see Note on page 95)
1½ tablespoons pine nuts

1. Preheat the oven to 350°F (180°C).
2. Heat the olive oil in a large skillet or saucepan over medium heat.
3. Add the onion and sauté for 5 minutes.
4. Add the garlic, mustard, thyme, herbal seasoning, black pepper, and a pinch of kosher salt, if desired, and the broccoli, mushrooms, and water. Sauté for an additional 5 minutes.
5. In a small bowl, mix the flour into the plant-based milk until smooth. Add to the broccoli mixture and cook for about 3 minutes, stirring occasionally, until the sauce is bubbly and thickened.
6. Pour the broccoli mixture into a 9-inch square baking dish.
7. Sprinkle with the plant-based cheese, bread crumbs, and pine nuts. Cover with foil and bake for 15 minutes. Remove the foil and bake for an additional 15 to 20 minutes, until tender and browned.

notes: You may use 12 ounces (340 g) of frozen broccoli, thawed and drained, in step 4. Reduce the cooking time to 2 minutes in step 4, and reduce the final baking time to 10 minutes in step 7.

For best results use white mushrooms; darker mushrooms can color the sauce.

variations: Substitute fresh green beans, sliced zucchini, or diced eggplant for the broccoli in step 4. You may need to adjust the cooking time—cook the vegetables until just tender. You may substitute walnuts, hazelnuts, or sunflower seeds for the pine nuts. To make this gluten-free, substitute 1½ tablespoons of cornstarch for the flour, use gluten-free bread crumbs, and check that all other ingredients are gluten-free.

> **PER SERVING:** 84 calories, 4 g protein, 9 g carbohydrate, 4 g fat, .5 g saturated fat,
> 3 g fiber, 2 g sugar, 52 mg sodium
> **STAR NUTRIENTS:** folate (15% DV), riboflavin (16% DV), thiamin (12% DV), vitamin C
> (37% DV), vitamin K (72% DV), calcium (11% DV), manganese (34% DV), potassium (11% DV)

See photo
on page 290

portobello mushroom and spinach pie

ACTIVE PREPARATION TIME: 27 minutes • TOTAL PREPARATION TIME: 1 hour 15 minutes

You won't believe that this rich, flavorful quiche is completely plant-based. It owes its creamy texture to tofu, and its savory, meaty flavor and texture to mushrooms and spinach. Serve this nutrient-rich pie for dinner with a salad, such as Summer Succotash with Heirloom Tomatoes (page 258), or for brunch with a side of seasonal fruit.

MAKES 8 SERVINGS
(one-eighth pie each)

Crust
1¼ cups (150 g) whole wheat pastry flour
1 tablespoon ground flaxseeds
¼ cup (50 ml) extra virgin olive oil
¼ cup (50 ml) unsweetened plain plant-based milk

Filling
½ tablespoon extra virgin olive oil
1 medium onion, diced
2 medium garlic cloves, minced
¼ teaspoon freshly ground black pepper
½ teaspoon dried mustard
2 tablespoons chopped fresh thyme, or 1½ teaspoons dried
1½ cups (105 g) sliced portobello mushrooms
5 ounces (142 g) fresh baby spinach leaves (4 cups tightly packed)
One 12-ounce (340 g) package extra firm tofu, drained and cubed
½ cup (119 ml) unsweetened plain plant-based milk
½ teaspoon nutmeg
Pinch of crushed red pepper
½ teaspoon turmeric
1 tablespoon nutritional yeast (see Note)
1 teaspoon vegan Worcestershire sauce (see Notes)
Pinch of sea salt, optional

Toppings
2 tablespoons whole grain bread crumbs (see Note on page 95)
½ cup shredded plant-based cheese, optional
1½ teaspoons chopped fresh thyme, or ½ teaspoon dried

1. Preheat the oven to 375°F (190°C).

2. To make the crust, mix the flour, flaxseeds, olive oil, and plant-based milk together to form a dough. Roll out on a lightly floured surface into a round crust slightly larger than 9 inches across. Fit into a 9-inch pie pan. Pierce all over with a fork and bake for 10 minutes.

3. Meanwhile, to make the filling, heat the olive oil in a large skillet over medium heat. Add the onion and sauté for 3 minutes. Add the garlic, black pepper, mustard, thyme, and mushrooms, and sauté for 3 additional minutes.

4. Add the spinach and sauté for about 2 minutes, just until wilted. Remove the pan from the heat.

5. Combine the tofu, plant-based milk, nutmeg, crushed red pepper, turmeric, nutritional yeast, Worcestershire sauce, and sea salt, if desired, in a blender and process until smooth, scraping down the sides as needed.

6. Stir the blended tofu into the spinach mixture in the skillet.

7. Fill the parbaked pie shell with the tofu filling. Bake for 30 minutes, uncovered. Sprinkle with the bread crumbs and cheese, return to the oven, and bake for an additional 15 to 20 minutes, until the top is golden and filling is firm.

8. Remove from the oven and garnish with the thyme. Slice into 8 servings.

notes: Nutritional yeast is an inactive yeast naturally rich in vitamins and minerals and often enriched with others (such as vitamin B). Because of its "cheesy" taste and nutritional profile, it is often used as a condiment in savory plant-based dishes.

You can find vegan Worcestershire sauce in gourmet and natural food stores.

variations: Substitute other greens for the spinach, such as dandelion, collard, or mustard greens. To make this gluten-free, replace the whole wheat pastry flour with 1 cup plus 2 tablespoons gluten-free flour blend (such as Bob's Red Mill or King Arthur Flour), use gluten-free bread crumbs, and check that all other ingredients are gluten-free.

PER SERVING: 222 calories, 9 g protein, 22 g carbohydrate, 11.5 g fat, 1.5 g saturated fat, 5 g fiber, 1 g sugar, 34 mg sodium
STAR NUTRIENTS: folate (14% DV), pantothenic acid (10% DV), thiamin (32% DV), vitamin A (41% DV), vitamin C (11% DV), vitamin K (272% DV), calcium (21% DV), iron (15% DV), magnesium (17% DV), potassium (11% DV)

Kiwi Herb Salad with Pistachios and Orange Dressing

Take a bite out of raw plant foods.

Spring Vegetable Salad with Green Goddess Dressing
Kiwi Herb Salad with Pistachios and Orange Dressing

Peppery arugula, crisp jicama, succulent peaches—these are but a few of the plants that taste their absolute best when eaten raw. Without heat to break down the plants' cell walls, their crunchy texture remains. And without cooking liquids to drain away fragrance and flavor molecules, these persist intact as you bite into the delicious vegetable or fruit. There's no doubt that one of the most sensual ways to enjoy plants is au naturel, without the aid of pots and pans. Don't even think about cooking a fresh, ripe strawberry in June, or tender leaves of spinach fresh from the garden in September.

Along with flavor, raw vegetables can have nutritional advantages. Cooking plant foods at high temperature, especially in water, can damage some sensitive nutrients, such as vitamins C and B. However, not all plants are best consumed raw. When you cook legumes and grains, you make their nutrients digestible. Some fruits and vegetables also benefit from heat, such as tomatoes, which provide more of the antioxidant lycopene when they are heated, because the plant walls open up to release it more effectively.

There is insufficient evidence to indicate you need to eat *only* raw foods, as some people propose. But it is a good idea to put more raw foods on the menu as another delicious way to celebrate plants. Here are a few of my personal raw favorites: vibrantly colored radishes and sweet bell pepper strips as an appetizer; "sandwiches" of basil, heirloom tomato, and avocado slices; ribbons of vegetables, such as cucumbers, broccoli, and carrots, created with a vegetable peeler (see page 158); a mixed greens salad topped with nectarine wedges; handfuls of fresh herbs, like parsley and cilantro, mixed into slaws or used as generous garnishes; and raw nut butter slathered over crisp apple slices.

spring vegetable salad with green goddess dressing

ACTIVE PREPARATION TIME: **20 minutes** • TOTAL PREPARATION TIME: **20 minutes**

The colors of this lovely raw spring salad—mint green, jade, lavender, rose red, sunny yellow—radiate spring joy. By serving vegetables in the raw— you won't lose a bit of their gorgeous, vibrant colors and crunchy textures. The portrait-perfect shades of this salad are accented with a healthy, plant-powered take on a retro favorite—green goddess dressing, which is founded on avocado, cucumbers, and dill.

MAKES 8 SERVINGS
(about 1¼ cups each)

Dressing
¼ cup (57 g) unsweetened plain cultured coconut yogurt
½ ripe medium avocado, peeled and diced
¼ cup (26 g) diced cucumber, with peel
¼ cup (15 g) chopped fresh dill, or 1 teaspoon dried
1 green onion, white and green parts, diced
1 medium garlic clove, minced
¼ teaspoon crushed red pepper
1 teaspoon white balsamic vinegar
1 tablespoon lemon juice

Salad
3 cups (108 g) baby salad greens
½ medium English cucumber
6 small radishes, quartered
1 cup (148 g) red cherry tomatoes
1½ cups (150 g) small fresh cauliflower florets, preferably purple (see Note)
1 cup (91 g) small fresh broccoli florets
½ medium yellow bell pepper, coarsely chopped
Fresh dill for garnish, optional

1. To make the dressing, add all the dressing ingredients to a blender and process until smooth. Scrape down the sides halfway through processing if needed.
2. To assemble the salad, line a platter or shallow bowl with the greens. Score the outside of the cucumber peel lengthwise with a fork to create shallow grooves. Slice thinly. Arrange all of the vegetables over the lettuce.
3. Pour the dressing over the salad (or serve on the side) and garnish with the fresh dill, if desired.

note: If purple cauliflower is not available, use white, orange, or green.

PER SERVING: 97 calories, 4 g protein, 17 g carbohydrate, 3 g fat, .5 g saturated fat, 7 g fiber, 9 g sugar, 21 mg sodium

STAR NUTRIENTS: folate (32% DV), vitamin A (30% DV), vitamin B6 (16% DV), vitamin C (151% DV), vitamin K (45% DV), calcium (14% DV), copper (19% DV), iron (14% DV), magnesium (17% DV), molybdenum (17% DV), phosphorus (12% DV), potassium (27% DV)

See photo
on page 298

kiwi herb salad with pistachios and orange dressing

ACTIVE PREPARATION TIME: **7 minutes** • TOTAL PREPARATION TIME: **7 minutes**

I love the combination of fresh fruits and vegetables in a salad—the sweet, fragrant flesh of fruits juxtaposed against the earthy, crisp vegetables. These raw ingredients are off the charts in the antioxidant vitamin C, which is delicate and easily damaged in cooking. Make a point of putting something raw—crunchy, fresh, and whole—on your menu every day.

MAKES 4 SERVINGS
(about 1¼ cups each)

3 cups (108 g) assorted herbs and salad greens (see Note)
2 medium fresh kiwis, peeled and sliced (see Note)
½ medium yellow bell pepper, sliced
2 tablespoons orange juice
2 teaspoons extra virgin olive oil
Freshly ground black pepper, to taste
½ teaspoon orange zest
Pinch of sea salt, optional
3 tablespoons roughly chopped raw pistachios

1. In a salad bowl, lightly toss together herbs and greens, kiwis, and bell pepper.

2. In a small dish, make the dressing by whisking together the orange juice, olive oil, black pepper, orange zest, and sea salt, if desired.

3. Drizzle the dressing over the salad and toss together. Sprinkle with the pistachios.

note: You may use pretrimmed, prewashed herbs and salad greens in a bag, and/or substitute fresh strawberries for the kiwis.

PER SERVING: 94 calories, 3 g protein, 10 g carbohydrate, 5 g fat, 1 g saturated fat, 3 g fiber, 4 g sugar, 58 mg sodium
STAR NUTRIENTS: vitamin A (43% DV), vitamin C (152% DV), vitamin K (17% DV)

Make it coffee or tea time today.

Lemon-Lavender Cooler
Whipped Hazelnut Iced Coffee
Flower and Pomegranate Tea

If there's one thing as clear as water, it's the fact that we are drinking too many sodas, sports drinks, and juice drinks in its place. The gallons we guzzle every year are doing significant damage to our health; new studies have linked the intake of high-sugar, high-calorie, zero-nutrient beverages to obesity, as well as type 2 diabetes and heart disease. A twelve-ounce soda contains *ten teaspoons* of sugar, so drinking it can produce an undesirable impact on your blood glucose, while adding about 150 calories to your day. These calories provide no nutrients, and they don't even fill you up!

So what *should* you be sipping? While your first choice should be water—straight from the tap (filtered is best)—your second choice should be a simple plant-powered beverage, like coffee and tea. These brews have been consumed for thousands of years in all corners of the globe. Even centuries ago, people believed coffee and tea could treat ailments and boost performance. And, as is true in so many cases, the old folk healers seem to have had it right. Coffee, made from the powerful *coffea* bean, and tea, made from the equally potent *Camellia senensis* leaf, are high in antioxidant and anti-inflammatory properties. Drinking coffee may protect you from type 2 diabetes, liver conditions, and colon cancer, in addition to boosting your mental and athletic performance; and tea can defend you from heart disease, cancer, and maybe even bone disease.

Both coffee and true tea contain caffeine, a natural stimulant that may be connected with some of its health benefits. If you experience problems such as insomnia and anxiety related to caffeine intake, you can still gain the antioxidant and anti-inflammatory benefits from decaffeinated versions of these plant beverages. All true teas—including black tea, made from mature, oxidized tea leaves; green tea made of mature, unoxidized tea leaves; and white tea, made from buds of tea—contain varying levels of antioxidant activity, so you can feel good about drinking the tea you like the best. While herbal teas are not "true" tea, they possess their own unique benefits, such as antioxidant and antimicrobial action.

So go ahead, drink tea and coffee for hydration and health. Just don't ruin your best intentions by drowning your cups with sugar, cream, and artificial ingredients. Try a splash of soy or almond milk, and a drizzle of agave if you prefer a hint of sweetness in your tea or coffee cup.

lemon-lavender cooler

ACTIVE PREPARATION TIME: **5 minutes** • TOTAL PREPARATION TIME: **1 hour 5 minutes**

On hot summer days, I love brewing up eclectic combinations of herbal teas to blend with freshly squeezed lemon or lime straight from the tree. The sun-kissed scents of lavender and lemon play together in this cooler. Serve it with a sprig of fresh lavender—a wonderful ingredient easy to grow in most locales—for a truly memorable, refreshing beverage.

MAKES 4 SERVINGS
(1 cup each)

4 cups (948 ml) hot water
3 lavender tea bags
Juice of 1 medium lemon
1 tablespoon honey or agave nectar
4 lemon slices
4 fresh lavender stems, optional

1. Combine the water and tea bags in a glass or ceramic pitcher. Let steep for 1 hour at room temperature.

2. Remove the tea bags and stir in the lemon juice and honey. Fill four glasses with ice cubes and add one cup of tea per glass.

3. Float the lemon slices and clean fresh lavender stems, if desired, on top.

note: You may brew the tea and store it in refrigerator for 3 to 4 days.

variation: Substitute mint tea and fresh mint for the lavender to make a Lemon-Mint Cooler.

PER SERVING: 23 calories, .5 g protein, 8 g carbohydrate, 0 g fat, 0 g saturated fat, 0 g fiber, 5 g sugar, 8 mg sodium
STAR NUTRIENTS: vitamin C (55% DV)

whipped hazelnut iced coffee

ACTIVE PREPARATION TIME: **6 minutes** • TOTAL PREPARATION TIME: **6 minutes**

Skip coffee shop frozen coffee concoctions—save money and calories by making your own plant-powered iced coffee, with the sweet, nutty taste of hazelnuts. And reap the rewards of coffee consumption—better performance and glucose control—with this wholesome, plant-powered beverage, done right.

MAKES 2 SERVINGS
(about 1 ⅓ cups each)

½ cup (119 g) brewed espresso
10 ice cubes
1 cup (237 ml) unsweetened hazelnut milk
1 teaspoon agave nectar
3 tablespoons hazelnuts
Pinch of allspice
Pinch of cocoa powder

1. Combine the espresso, ice cubes, milk, agave, and hazelnuts in a blender. Process for 1 to 2 minutes, until the contents are very smooth. The nuts require extra processing for smoothness.

2. Pour into two mugs and sprinkle with a pinch of allspice and cocoa powder.

variation: Substitute almond milk and almonds for the hazelnut milk and hazelnuts.

PER SERVING: 115 calories, 2 g protein, 14 g carbohydrate, 6 g fat, 0 g saturated fat, 1 g fiber, 10 g sugar, 68 mg sodium
STAR NUTRIENTS: niacin (16% DV), riboflavin (10% DV), calcium (30% DV), copper (15% DV), magnesium (15% DV), manganese (32% DV), potassium (10% DV)

flower and pomegranate tea

ACTIVE PREPARATION TIME: **4 minutes** • TOTAL PREPARATION TIME: **18 minutes**

You can't beat freshly brewed teas for plant-powered hydration. These brews are packed with antioxidant and anti-inflammatory action, sans the artificial ingredients and sugar, if you make them at home. In my flower tea, I add an enchanting touch of edible flowers in tandem with hibiscus and rose tea and pomegranate juice to create an aromatic, pretty beverage that is sure to turn heads at your next brunch or luncheon.

MAKES 4 SERVINGS
(1¼ cups each)

4 cups (948 ml) boiling water
2 hibiscus herbal tea bags (see Notes)
1 rose herbal tea bag (see Notes)
1 cup (237 ml) pomegranate juice
12 ice cubes, optional
Edible flowers (e.g., pansies, nasturtium, and lavender), optional

1. Pour the boiling water into a glass pitcher. Add the tea bags and allow to steep for at least 15 minutes.
2. Remove the tea bags and add the pomegranate juice.
3. Fill four glasses with the ice cubes and the tea (or chill the pitcher in the refrigerator until serving time). Float edible flowers on top of the tea in each glass, if desired, and serve immediately.

notes: You may use sweet rose or rose hips tea, as well as other tea blends, including lemon rose or raspberry rose.

You can find edible flowers in some natural and gourmet food stores, or you can harvest these from your own flower garden. Just be sure to use those that are not treated with pesticides or fertilizers and wash them well.

variation: Substitute peach or cranberry juice for the pomegranate juice.

PER SERVING: 32 calories, 0 g protein, 8 g carbohydrate, 0 g fat, 0 g saturated fat, 0 g fiber, 6 g sugar, 12 mg sodium

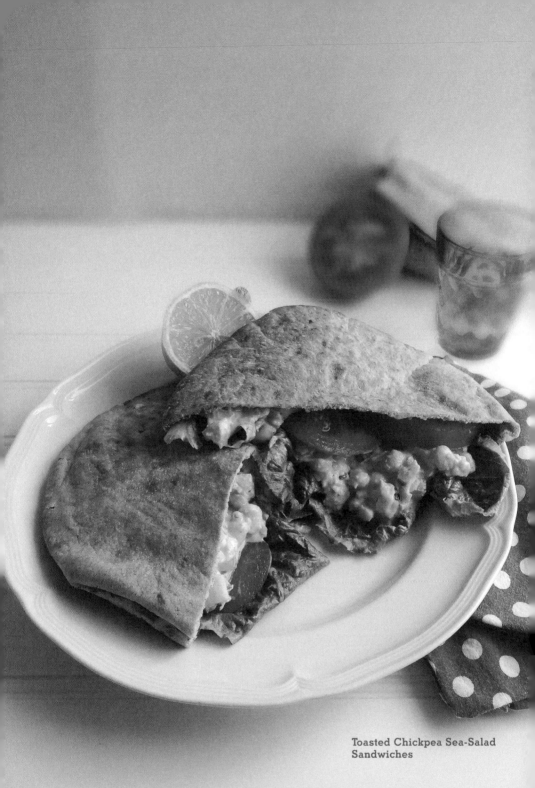

Toasted Chickpea Sea-Salad
Sandwiches

Find a place for fermented foods.

Korean Kimchi Hot Pot

Toasted Chickpea Sea-Salad Sandwiches

Long before refrigerators and freezers, even before canning, people had to find ways to preserve nature's bounty to last through the lean times. As ingenuous and tenacious as we humans were, we discovered fermentation. Of course, fermentation, the process of converting sugar in foods into acids, gases, or alcohol, had been around long before we were, but our ancestors found a way to capture and control it.

During this process, microorganisms such as yeasts and bacteria, which occur naturally in the environment or are introduced into foods, work their magic altering foods. Fermentation turns milk into yogurt, grape juice into wine, and cucumbers into pickles.

All over the world, traditional fermented foods are part of the culinary fabric. German sauerkraut, Korean kimchi (cabbage), Ethiopian injeera (teff flatbread), Indonesian tempeh (fermented grain and soy cakes), Japanese natto (soybeans), and Polynesian poi (taro) are just a few examples of classic fermented cultural foods. These foods provide us more than just explosive taste (and alcoholic buzz, in the case of wine and beer). Fermentation breaks down food, which may make certain nutrients more digestible. And it also introduces beneficial bacteria—probiotics—into your intestinal tract, which can provide a number of benefits, ranging from immune support to better digestive health.

Unfortunately, many foods that were traditionally fermented, such as pickles and sauerkraut, are now produced within the modern industrial food setting, where vinegar and canning have taken the place of live bacteria. While they are still plant-based foods (although often very high in salt), these industrialized versions are not created under the age-old fermentation principles of introducing microorganisms into foods. But true fermented foods have continued to be produced and are now experiencing something of a renaissance: pickles, kombucha (a fermented beverage), kimchi, and more are increasingly available in markets. Look for "contains live cultures" on the label as a sign. You can even make your own fermented foods, such as yogurt, sourdough bread, and pickles. Take a lesson from the history books and find a place for more fermented foods in your diet.

korean kimchi hot pot

ACTIVE PREPARATION TIME: **23 minutes** • TOTAL PREPARATION TIME: **28 minutes**

Kimchi is a traditional fermented dish in Korea. Made of vegetables such as cabbage and radishes and flavored with red chiles, kimchi is one of the most famous examples of pickled vegetables, dating all the way back to the tenth century BC. Fermentation was born out of necessity to preserve foods, but we now know that the introduction of natural bacteria into foods like kimchi offers myriad health rewards. The sour, crisp bite of kimchi is the hallmark of this delectable hot pot.

MAKES 6 SERVINGS
(1 cup soup with ½ cup noodles each)

1 tablespoon sesame oil
1 medium carrot, sliced
2 medium garlic cloves, minced
2 cups (140 g) Chinese (or Napa) cabbage, thinly sliced
1½ cups (105 g) sliced mushrooms (e.g., button, shitake, or oyster)
One 14-ounce (397 g) jar spicy vegetarian kimchi, with liquid (see Notes)
½ tablespoon kochujang paste (also known as gochujang; see Notes)
1 tablespoon reduced sodium soy sauce
2½ cups (593 ml) water
One 14-ounce (397 g) package extra firm tofu, drained and sliced into strips (pressed, for best results—see page 103)
4 medium green onions, white and green parts, sliced
One 9.5-ounce (270 g) package plain ramen noodles, uncooked

1. Heat the sesame oil in a large skillet or wok over medium heat. Add the carrot and stir-fry for 4 minutes.
2. Add the garlic and cabbage and stir-fry for an additional 2 minutes.
3. Add the mushrooms and stir-fry for an additional 3 minutes.
4. Add the kimchi (including liquid), kochujang paste, soy sauce, and water. Stir well and simmer for 8 minutes. Add the tofu and green onions and simmer for an additional 2 minutes.
5. Meanwhile, bring a medium pot of water to a boil over high heat. Add the ramen and cook on medium heat for 4 minutes (or according to the package directions)—do not overcook. Drain immediately, rinse, return to the pot, and cover to keep warm.
6. To serve, dish up ½ cup of noodles each into six large soup bowls. Ladle 1 cup of kimchi mixture over the noodles. Serve immediately.

notes: Fermented vegetarian kimchi (such as King's Spicy Kimchi) is available in specialty stores. When you open the jar, the fermentation may cause bubbling and possible leaking over the jar.

Kochujang paste is a hot pepper paste available in Asian markets and online.

variation: To make this dish gluten-free, substitute rice noodles for the ramen and cook according to package directions. Ensure the soy sauce and all other ingredients used are gluten-free.

PER SERVING: 262 calories, 15 g protein, 37 g carbohydrate, 6 g fat, 1 g saturated fat, 5 g fiber, 3 g sugar, 182 mg sodium
STAR NUTRIENTS: folate (33% DV), niacin (19% DV), riboflavin (15% DV), thiamin (23% DV), vitamin A (102% DV), vitamin C (63% DV), vitamin K (45% DV), calcium (20% DV), iron (19% DV), magnesium (11% DV)

See photo
on page 308

toasted chickpea sea-salad sandwiches

ACTIVE PREPARATION TIME: 26 minutes • TOTAL PREPARATION TIME: 26 minutes

Flavored with sea vegetables and fermented pickles, this chickpea-based sandwich filling is a perfect plant-powered replacement for tuna salad in sandwiches and green salads. Rich in protein, fiber, and other essential nutrients, this salad also provides a helping of healthy bacteria, compliments of the fermented pickles—they possess live bacteria and are increasingly available in natural food stores.

MAKES 6 SERVINGS
(1 sandwich each)

12 slices of whole grain bread (e.g., rye, whole wheat, gluten-free multigrain; see Notes)
One 15-ounce (425 g) can chickpeas, no salt added, rinsed and drained (or 1¾ cups cooked)
¼ cup (25 g) finely diced celery
2 tablespoons finely diced white onion
⅓ cup (52 g) finely diced fresh fermented pickles (with live active cultures)
1 medium carrot, shredded
2 tablespoons chopped fresh parsley
1 tablespoon capers, rinsed and chopped
2 tablespoons finely sliced dried seaweed (e.g., nori, arame)
3 tablespoons reduced-fat plant-based mayonnaise (see page 343)
½ teaspoon prepared yellow mustard
½ teaspoon miso paste (see Note on page 249)
1 tablespoon fresh lemon juice
½ teaspoon reduced sodium soy sauce
½ teaspoon nutritional yeast (see Note on page 161)

Toppings
6 romaine lettuce leaves
2 medium tomatoes, sliced
12 slices fresh fermented pickles, drained

1. Preheat the oven to 375°F (190°C). Arrange the bread on a baking sheet and toast in the oven for 5 to 8 minutes, until lightly browned, or use a toaster.
2. Meanwhile, in a medium bowl, mash the chickpeas with a potato masher into a chunky paste.
3. Mix in the celery, onion, pickles, carrot, parsley, capers, and seaweed.

4. In a small bowl, make the dressing by mixing together the plant-based mayonnaise, mustard, miso paste, lemon juice, soy sauce, and nutritional yeast until smooth.

5. Stir the dressing into the chickpea mixture.

6. To make a sandwich, spread ½ cup of the filling across 1 slice of toasted bread. Top with 1 lettuce leaf, 2 slices of tomato, and 2 additional pickle slices. Top with another slice of bread. Continue until you have 6 sandwiches. Slice them in half diagonally and serve immediately.

notes: You may substitute a whole grain pita half or buns for the bread, or omit the bread and serve the salad on a bed of lettuce greens.

If you do not plan on making all of the sandwiches at one time, make only the sandwiches desired and store the leftover filling in an airtight container in the refrigerator for up to 3 days.

PER SERVING: 395 calories, 15 g protein, 67 g carbohydrate, 9 g fat, 2 g saturated fat, 9 g fiber, 10 g sugar, 623 mg sodium
STAR NUTRIENTS: folate (18% DV), niacin (18% DV), riboflavin (11% DV), thiamin (21% DV), vitamin A (71% DV), vitamin B6 (13% DV), vitamin C (32% DV), vitamin K (87% DV), calcium (11% DV), copper (22% DV), iron (19% DV), magnesium (28% DV), manganese (10% DV), phosphorus (19% DV), potassium (16% DV), selenium (33% DV), zinc (14% DV)

Black Bean Brownies with Walnuts

Splurge on dark chocolate in petite portions.

Chile Hot Chocolate
Black Bean Brownies with Walnuts

I can remember the days when giving in to your chocolate craving was something you felt guilty about. Have those days ever gone by the wayside! Chocolate—particularly dark chocolate—now has a health halo, thanks to its polyphenols, which act as antioxidants. Studies show that if you indulge in a small amount (1 ounce) of daily dark chocolate, you can protect your heart by maintaining healthy blood vessels, preventing blood clots, and lowering blood pressure, inflammation, and cholesterol levels.

Many times, the lessons we learn about good nutrition point us straight back to eating plants as nature made them, and chocolate is a perfect example. Originating in the Amazon, cocoa beans grow on cacao trees that flourish in tropical locations. The ancient Mayans and Aztecs, who consumed cocoa beans in a bitter, unsweetened brew or porridge, believed it to be a health elixir. Considering that 10 percent of the total weight of cocoa powder is made up of polyphenols, it looks like they were right. Spaniards discovered the secret of chocolate along their quest in the New World but transformed cocoa in the sixteenth century into a mixture of refined sugar and ground cocoa beans—a foreshadow of modern-day chocolate. And the rest is history.

Of course, today's chocolate bars, blended with a number of other ingredients, such as fats, milk, emulsifiers, and sugar, are nothing like the simple concoctions consumed in the jungles thousands of years ago. In order to gain the health benefits of eating chocolate, you need to be choosy. Find a dark chocolate bar that has at least 70 percent cocoa content; avoid milk chocolate, which has very low percentages of cocoa, and white chocolate, which has none. Read the ingredients list to see what you're getting—ideally few added sugars, and cocoa butter rather than hydrogenated oils. Limit yourself to just an ounce a day as a special treat (see page 221), or a small amount of cocoa in smoothies, breads, and cookies. And don't forget to consider how the cocoa beans were grown for your chocolate bar. We vote with our dollars, so if you can afford it, always pick organic and fairly traded cocoa beans.

chile hot chocolate

Cocoa beans were discovered by the Mayans centuries ago, so this beverage—infused with the flavors of chile de árbol, dark chocolate, and agave—is in their honor. These tastes blend into a rich, creamy dairy-free beverage, with a hint of heat. Stir up a pot after a blustery winter day for a dose of antioxidants that will soothe both your body and soul.

MAKES 2 SERVINGS
(about ¾ cup each)

1 small dried *chile de árbol* (see Notes)
1½ cups (356 g) unsweetened plain plant-based milk
2 cinnamon sticks
2 ounces (57 g) dark chocolate (at least 70% cocoa), coarsely
    grated or chopped (see Notes)
1 tablespoon agave nectar

1. Place a small pot over medium heat. Add the chile de árbol and cook for about 1 minute, until it begins to change color.
2. Remove the chile, let cool, and grind it (skin, seeds, and all) in a blender, small food processor, or spice grinder until ground.
3. Add the plant-based milk and cinnamon sticks to the same pot and heat over low heat for about 5 minutes, stirring occasionally, until the mixture is hot and bubbly. Remove the cinnamon sticks and reserve.
4. Add the chocolate, agave, and ground chile (as much as desired), stirring vigorously with a wire whisk until the chocolate is melted and the mixture is foamy.
5. Divide the hot chocolate between two mugs or cups, and serve with the cinnamon sticks.

notes: Chile de arbol is a small potent chile often found dried in Latin markets, as well as many supermarkets.

For best results, use Mexican dark chocolate, such as Cortés or Ibarra.

PER SERVING: 242 calories, 7 g protein, 28 g carbohydrate, 11 g fat, 6 g saturated fat, 3 g fiber, 23 g sugar, 102 mg sodium
STAR NUTRIENTS: riboflavin (24% DV), thiamin (19% DV), calcium (23% DV), iron (12% DV), magnesium (15% DV)

black bean brownies with walnuts

See photo
on page 314

ACTIVE PREPARATION TIME: **9 minutes** • TOTAL PREPARATION TIME: **54 minutes**

*Here's the perfect scenario—a dense, moist brownie packed with cocoa
polyphenols and bean nutrition—protein, fiber, and even antioxidants! The
beans replace the grains and some of the fat in this gluten-free, egg-free
brownie. I guarantee that nobody will guess the magic ingredient—black
beans—in this delicious treat. What a great way to get kids (and grown-
ups!) to eat their beans.*

MAKES 16 SERVINGS
(one 2 by 2-inch brownie each)

Nonstick cooking spray
One 15-ounce (425 g) can black beans, no salt added, rinsed
    and drained (or 1¾ cups cooked)
½ cup (170 g) honey or agave nectar
½ cup (43 g) unsweetened cocoa powder
2 tablespoons chia seeds (see Notes on page 139)
1 teaspoon pure vanilla extract
3 tablespoons canola oil, expeller pressed
½ teaspoon baking powder
½ cup (85 g) dairy-free, dark chocolate chips
½ cup (58 g) chopped walnuts

1. Preheat the oven to 350°F (180°C). Spray an 8 by 8-inch baking dish
with nonstick cooking spray.
2. Place the black beans, honey, cocoa powder, chia seeds, vanilla, canola
oil, and baking powder in a blender. Process until smooth. Scrape down
the sides halfway through blending if needed.
3. Pour the batter into the prepared baking dish.
4. Sprinkle the chocolate chips and walnuts evenly across the top of the
brownies.
5. Bake for 45 to 50 minutes, until the edges pull away from the side of the
pan and the brownies are firm.
6. Cool for a few minutes, and then slice into 16 squares.

note: This makes a chewy, moist brownie.

PER SERVING: 149 calories, 3 g protein, 20 g carbohyrate, 8 g fat, 2 g saturated fat,
3 g fiber, 11 g sugar, 99 mg sodium
STAR NUTRIENTS: magnesium (10% DV), manganese (14% DV)

Splurge on dark chocolate in petite portions. • 317

Zucchini Verde
Sprouted Rice

Give sprouted grains (and legumes) a try.

Zucchini Verde Sprouted Rice
Sprouted Lentil Granola with Apricots

❦

Each whole grain kernel and legume is essentially a seed, waiting to sprout and give life to a brand-new tiny plant. That's why seeds are packed with such rich nutrients: they must support the new baby grass that will burst forth and flourish. All you've got to do is give that whole grain kernel a little moisture and warmth, and voilà—you have a sprouted (or "germinated") grain. The same is true of legumes.

Sprouted grains and legumes are all the rage. Just walk through a natural food store and you will see bags and bins with a variety of sprouted kernels. I'm not talking about the fully sprouted seeds you find in the refrigerated section, such as alfalfa or bean sprouts, that sport inches of tender sprouts emerging from the seed (these are in essence the young plant: no longer a seed, but a grass in the case of alfalfa sprouts, or a bean plant in the case of bean sprouts). I'm referring to grains or legumes with just the slightest hint of a sprout emerging from their kernels. These are still seeds, but their little sprout is a calling card for changes that have occurred inside—changes that may benefit you when you eat them.

During the germination process, enzymes go to work on some of the nutrients in the kernel, making them more digestible when you eat them. And the sprouting process also pushes up levels of nutrients, like fiber, vitamins B and C, and calcium. You don't have to eat *only* sprouted grains and legumes for optimal health, but it's another way to celebrate the pleasures of eating whole plant-based foods. While you can find sprouted grains and legumes, such as sprouted rice, lentils, and wheat, in natural food stores, you can also sprout them at home. Just soak grains or legumes in water overnight, drain the water, cover the kernels with a damp cloth, place the bowl in a warm location, and rinse daily with fresh lukewarm water, until tiny sprouts of one to two millimeters emerge (in about one to three days). You can cook them up just like you would any whole grain, and their roughly milled whole grain flours are delicious in breads and baked goods.

See photo
on page 318

zucchini verde sprouted rice

ACTIVE PREPARATION TIME: **17 minutes** • TOTAL PREPARATION TIME: **1 hour**

This verdant Latin-inspired rice side dish is packed with the flavors of fresh cilantro, zucchini, bell pepper, green onions, and just a hint of jalapeño. It's the perfect dish to celebrate today's sprouted grains renaissance. Sprouting brown rice improves both its nutritional profile and its digestibility. I love to serve this colorful, nutritious rice with a Latin entrée, such as Pigeon Peas with Pumpkin and Sofrito (page 200).

MAKES 8 SERVINGS
(about ¾ cup each)

3¾ cups (889 ml) water
1½ cups (300 g) sprouted (or germinated) short grain brown rice
  (see Notes)
1 teaspoon reduced sodium vegetable broth base
½ tablespoon extra virgin olive oil
2 small zucchinis, diced
2 medium garlic cloves, minced
½ teaspoon cumin
½ medium green bell pepper, diced
3 medium green onions, white and green parts, sliced
1 small jalapeño pepper, seeded and quartered
1½ cups (90 g) loosely packed fresh cilantro
2 tablespoons lemon juice

1. Heat the water in a medium pot over high heat. Add the sprouted rice and broth base, cover, reduce the heat to medium, and cook 45 to 50 minutes, until tender.
2. Heat the olive oil in a large skillet or sauté pan over medium heat. Add the zucchinis, garlic, cumin, and bell pepper. Sauté for 5 minutes.
3. Add the cooked rice and green onions to the skillet and cook for an additional 4 minutes.
4. Meanwhile, combine the jalapeño, cilantro, and lemon juice in a blender or food processor and process until finely chopped but not liquefied.
5. Add the cilantro mixture to the rice, stir in well, and cook until just heated through, about 2 minutes.

notes: Look for sprouted grains, such as rice, in natural food stores or well-stocked supermarkets. If you can't find sprouted brown rice, you can sprout it yourself. This process works for every kind of grain and legume: Sort and rinse the grains or legumes, place in a bowl, cover with water and a clean cloth, and soak overnight in a warm place. Rinse in a sieve with warm, clean water, and return to the bowl, and repeat this process a couple of times a day for 1 to 3 days, until the grains or legumes show just the smallest hint of a sprout emerging from the kernel.

You can use a rice cooker for step 1, if desired.

variations: You may substitute sprouted quinoa, wheat berries, or rye berries in step 1, following appropriate amount of liquid and cooking time as indicated on package. You can also substitute regular brown rice for sprouted rice, if desired.

PER SERVING: 159 calories, 4 g protein, 31 g carbohydrate, 2 g fat, .0 g saturated fat, 3 g fiber, 3 g sugar, 157 mg sodium
STAR NUTRIENTS: niacin (11% DV), thiamin (13% DV), vitamin A (10% DV), vitamin B6 (19% DV), vitamin C (54% DV), vitamin K (29% DV), magnesium (17% DV), potassium (10% DV)

---

sprouted lentil granola with apricots

ACTIVE PREPARATION TIME: 18 minutes • TOTAL PREPARATION TIME: 45 minutes

Did you know that you can add legumes, such as these tiny sprouted lentils, to a number of baked goods? When baked, they add a dose of crunch—as well as protein and fiber—to this granola, which is flavored with apricots and baking spices. Make up a batch to sprinkle over plant-based yogurt, cereals, and fruits all week long.

MAKES 12 SERVINGS
(about ⅓ cup each)

1 cup (192 g) dried sprouted small lentils (green, yellow, red, or multicolored; see Note)
1½ cups (356 ml) water
2 cups (312 g) old-fashioned rolled oats
¼ cup (23 g) unsweetened shredded coconut
⅓ cup (47 g) sunflower seeds, hulled
2 tablespoons hemp seeds
2 tablespoons chia seeds
½ cup (74 g) chopped dates
½ cup (65 g) chopped dried apricots
2 tablespoons canola oil, expeller pressed
2 tablespoons maple syrup
2 teaspoons vanilla extract
½ teaspoon cinnamon
½ teaspoon allspice
½ teaspoon nutmeg
½ teaspoon cardamom

1. Add the lentils and water to a small pot, cover, and bring to a boil over high heat. Reduce the heat to medium and cook for just 10 minutes, keeping the lentils firm and slightly crunchy (do not overcook). Drain any remaining water and set the lentils aside.
2. Meanwhile, preheat the oven to 350°F (180°C).
3. In a large bowl, combine the oats, coconut, sunflower seeds, hemp seeds, chia seeds, dates, and apricots. Add the cooked lentils.
4. In a small pot, mix together the canola oil, maple syrup, vanilla, cinnamon, allspice, nutmeg, and cardamom. Bring to a boil over medium heat, stirring constantly. Remove from the heat and pour over the granola, stirring to combine well.
5. Spread the granola in a thin layer on a baking sheet. Bake for about 30 minutes, until golden brown. Stir every 10 minutes.
6. Store in an airtight container for up to one month.

note: If you cannot find sprouted lentils, make your own (see page 319) or use plain small lentils.

variations: Substitute sesame or pumpkin seeds for the sunflower seeds, and raisins, dried cherries, or chopped dried apples for the apricots.

PER SERVING: 171 calories, 4 g protein, 25 g carbohydrate, 7 g fat, 1 g saturated fat, 4 g fiber, 11 g sugar, 3 mg sodium
STAR NUTRIENTS: thiamin (11% DV), vitamin E (10% DV), copper (16% DV), iron (15% DV), manganese (26% DV)

50

Indulge moderately in alcohol, especially red wine.

Hot Spiced Wine with Raisins and Almonds

❧

Pour a glass of well-made wine and you will reveal a marvel. It came from grapes that were grown on a vine in a sunny vineyard, crushed into juice, fermented in a tank, and then perhaps aged in an oak barrel before the resulting wine was poured into a glass bottle, corked, and placed in a cool, moist cave for several months, maybe years. A whiff of wine might yield surprising aromas of jasmine, smoke, cedar, or tropical fruits. A taste might reveal even more flavors, such as sea salt, black pepper, strawberries, and chocolate, all of which arose naturally during the process of wine making.

Wine making is but another example of a plant-powered tradition that has brought health and pleasure to people throughout the centuries: it dates back at least ten thousand years! And now we know that moderate consumption of wine (one serving a day for women; two for men)—along with other alcohol, such as beer and spirits—offers some proven health benefits, especially for cardiovascular health. Moderate drinkers have half the risk of dying from coronary heart disease and stroke that nondrinkers have. In the case of red wine, these benefits may be traced back to hundreds of polyphenol compounds found in grape skins. And alcohol itself seems to protect the heart by improving blood cholesterol and preventing blood clots.

However, alcohol intake—even moderate—is a risk factor for developing cancer. The American Institute for Cancer Research now says that for cancer prevention, you should avoid alcohol, though it concedes that moderate intake has other health benefits that might make imbibing worthwhile, if you enjoy alcohol. Remember, any benefits from alcohol consumption quickly disappear if you drink heavily, which can cause disease and death. Therefore, the American Heart Association suggests that you shouldn't pick up drinking just to gain any potential benefits.

If you already enjoy alcohol, do so moderately. Drink like they do in the Mediterranean, where wine consumption is part of the much-heralded Mediterranean diet. Pour a glass of wine, and savor it in the company of good food, friends, and family.

hot spiced wine with raisins and almonds

ACTIVE PREPARATION TIME: **6 minutes** • TOTAL PREPARATION TIME: **2 hours 10 minutes**

In many northern European countries, a simple blend of wine, juice, and spices is served in the winter to warm you to the bone. And this beverage does a lot to warm the spirit, as well! A variation of this brew may be found everywhere from Swiss ski lodges on the snowy mountainside to the hearth of a Swedish home during the holiday season.

MAKES 6 SERVINGS
(about ½ cup each)

2 cups (474 ml) red wine (e.g., Merlot, Cabernet, Syrah)
1 cup (237 ml) cranberry-berry juice (see Notes)
1 tablespoon honey
1 teaspoon whole cloves
1 teaspoon whole allspice
2 cinnamon sticks
½ teaspoon orange zest
¼ cup (41 g) raisins
¼ cup (23 g) slivered almonds

1. Pour the red wine, juice, and honey into a small bowl.
2. Add the cloves, allspice, cinnamon sticks, and orange zest. Cover and let steep for 2 hours at room temperature.
3. Line a strainer with a paper towel and strain the wine mixture through it into a small pot. Discard the spices and zest.
4. Add the raisins and almonds to the wine and heat only until it begins steaming—do not boil.
5. Serve in small mugs.

notes: You may use cranberry-raspberry, cranberry-blueberry, or cranberry-strawberry juice.

This may be prepared ahead, refrigerated, and reheated just before serving. In that case, do not add the raisins or almonds until you're preparing to serve (step 4).

PER SERVING: 130 calories, 1 g protein, 13 g carbohydrate, 2 g fat, 0 g saturated fat, 1 g fiber, 9 g sugar, 8 mg sodium
STAR NUTRIENTS: vitamin C (20% DV), manganese (20% DV)

Carrot Spice Cupcakes with Chocolate
"Cream Cheese" Frosting

Share the plant-powered love!

Cashew Cheese with Popped Seeds
Butternut Squash and Caramelized Onion Salad
Carrot Spice Cupcakes with Chocolate "Cream Cheese" Frosting

As you've been acquiring your plant-powered habits, you've probably noticed how vibrant you feel, with an extra kick in your step and perhaps a better result in your latest checkup or a more favorable number on the scale. These benefits are all associated with a plant-based diet.

Now it's time to share this gift of well-being with your friends and family. It's easy; you can throw a plant-powered party and cook up some of your favorite recipes (the ones in this chapter make for a great spread). Start cooking these foods for dinner every night for your entire family, share them at picnics and holiday dinners, and pack them up to take along to the office.

As you learn more and more about savoring the flavors of whole plant foods, open your horizons to even more adventurous plant-centric living. For example, dive into vegetables from the sea—a whole underwater world of umami-packed plants, such as seaweed, sea palm, sea grapes, and more, which are rich in nutrients, such as vitamins, minerals, and anti-inflammatory compounds. Don't be afraid to try new, unusual plants wherever you find them. Visit farmers markets and ethnic supermarkets for produce finds like Asian vegetables, including bitter melon and Chinese celery, and Latin vegetables, including nopal and yuca root. Keep your eyes open for new spices and herbs, such as pungent long pepper and sumac. And try new grains and legumes, such as freekeh, the Middle Eastern roasted wheat grain, and chana dal, a small pea used in Indian cuisine. Let your enthusiasm for the flavors, textures, and wholesome qualities of plant foods bubble over and inspire others around you.

Start discovering plant-powered resources in your community, including local vegan or vegetarian restaurants, food shops, or cooking classes, and Meetup.com groups for vegetarian or vegan advocates. Take your newfound plant-based interests online and discover a plant-powered community through websites, organizations, and blogs. If you feel inspired, you could even chronicle your own plant-powered life experience by starting your own blog.

cashew cheese with popped seeds

ACTIVE PREPARATION TIME: **14 minutes** • TOTAL PREPARATION TIME: **14 minutes**
(not including soaking and chilling time)

Rejoice at your newfound plant-powered attitude and get ready to show-case it at your next potluck, party, or holiday celebration. Making your own vegan cheese is all the rage! Some plant-based cheeses are stunningly close to the original, complete with rinds, casings, and aged flavors. Perfecting them is a true artisanal skill that takes practice, but this soft, spreadable cashew cheese recipe is a simple way to get started. You don't need any special ingredients or equipment: just raw cashews and a few seasonings. Serve it with popped seeds to make the flavors, well, pop.

MAKES 8 SERVINGS
(1 ounce each)

Cashew Cheese
1 cup (137 g) raw cashews
1 tablespoon extra virgin olive oil
¼ cup (119 ml) lemon juice
3 tablespoons water
1 teaspoon nutritional yeast
¼ teaspoon turmeric
Pinch of kosher salt, optional

Popped Seeds
1 teaspoon extra virgin olive oil
½ teaspoon cumin seeds
½ teaspoon mustard seeds
½ teaspoon coriander seeds

1. Place the cashews in a bowl and cover with water. Cover with a towel and soak overnight at room temperature.

2. The next day, drain the cashews and rinse well in cool water.

3. Add the soaked, drained cashews, olive oil, lemon juice, water, nutritional yeast, turmeric, and a pinch of kosher salt, if desired, to a blender or food processor.

4. Process the cashew mixture for about 2 minutes, until very smooth and creamy. Scrape down the sides of container during processing if necessary.

5. Line a strainer or colander with cheesecloth or a clean dish towel and place it over a bowl. Pour the cashew mixture into the lined strainer, then cover tightly with the cheesecloth or towel. Let stand at room temperature for 4 hours.

6. Unfold the cheesecloth or towel and carefully transfer the cashew cheese to another clean cheesecloth or towel. Wrap up the cashew cheese and place in the refrigerator overnight (or for at least 8 hours).

7. Unfold the towel and shape the soft cashew cheese into a small round loaf.

8. To make the popped seeds, just before serving, heat the olive oil in a small skillet over medium-high heat. Add the seeds and stir for about 1 minute until they pop.

9. Place the cashew cheese on a serving container and drizzle with the hot popped seeds and oil. Serve immediately.

notes: You may skip the seeds in step 8 if you prefer a simple, soft cashew cheese.

This cheese is not firm enough to shred or slice thinly, but you can slice it into slabs for sandwiches or spread it on crackers.

Store in the refrigerator for up to one week.

PER SERVING: 120 calories, 3 g protein, 6 g carbohydrate, 10 g fat, 1.5 g saturated fat, 1 g fiber, 1 g sugar, 4 mg sodium

STAR NUTRIENTS: copper (19% DV), magnesium (13% DV), manganese (15% DV), phosphorus (10% DV)

butternut squash and caramelized onion salad

ACTIVE PREPARATION TIME: **12 minutes** • TOTAL PREPARATION TIME: **51 minutes**

Now that your cup overflows with plant-powered joy, it's time to share it! The best way to show off the power of plants is through flavorful, gorgeous dishes, such as this fall-time favorite. The caramelized onion and baking spices blend with roasted butternut squash—off the charts with eye-loving vitamin A—for a beautiful and comforting salad experience. If you're in a rush, use prechopped butternut squash, available in many supermarkets.

MAKES 4 SERVINGS
(about 1¼ cup each)

1 tablespoon extra virgin olive oil
1 tablespoon maple syrup
1 tablespoon orange juice
1 teaspoon white wine vinegar
Pinch of freshly ground black pepper
½ teaspoon pumpkin pie spice
Pinch of sea salt, optional
12 ounces (340 g or 2½ cups) peeled and chopped butternut
    squash
½ medium yellow onion, thinly sliced
¼ cup (32 g) shelled pumpkin seeds
3 cups (170 g) baby salad greens with radicchio

1. Preheat the oven to 375°F (190°C).
2. In a small dish, make the dressing by whisking together the olive oil, maple syrup, orange juice, vinegar, black pepper, and pumpkin pie spice. Taste and add a pinch of sea salt, if desired.
3. Combine the squash, onion, and pumpkin seeds in a shallow baking dish.
4. Pour the dressing over the squash mixture and toss together.
5. Place the baking dish on the top rack of the oven and bake for about 40 minutes, until the vegetables are tender and the onions are brown.
6. Remove the dish from the oven and let cool until room temperature.
7. Fill a salad bowl (or line a serving plate) with the salad greens and radicchio. Top with cooled squash mixture and toss together. Serve immediately.

variations: Substitute another winter squash, such as carnival, acorn, or turban, for the butternut. Substitute another lettuce blend, such as baby spinach, kale, or arugula.

PER SERVING: 132 calories, 3 g protein, 21 g carbohydrate, 5 g fat, 1 g saturated fat, 4 g fiber, 7 g sugar, 21 mg sodium
STAR NUTRIENTS: vitamin A (211% DV), vitamin C (34% DV), magnesium (13% DV), manganese (21% DV), potassium (12% DV)

See photo on page 326

carrot spice cupcakes with chocolate "cream cheese" frosting

ACTIVE PREPARATION TIME: **26 minutes** • TOTAL PREPARATION TIME: **1 hour 15 minutes**

Who says treats can't be both wholesome and delicious? Case in point: my plant-powered, whole grain, vegan cupcakes—naturally sweetened with a touch of agave nectar and raisins, and chock-full of shredded carrots and baking spices. Bake them up for dessert, coffee breaks, and bagged lunches.

MAKES 12 SERVINGS
(1 cupcake each)

⅓ cup (79 ml) canola oil, expeller pressed
1 teaspoon vanilla extract
1 cup (237 ml) plain, unsweetened plant-based milk
⅓ cup (113 g) honey or agave nectar
1 tablespoon ground flaxseeds
2 tablespoons chia seeds (see Notes on page 139)
1¾ cups (193 g) shredded carrots (about 3 medium)
2 cups (240 g) white whole wheat flour
1 teaspoon baking powder
1 teaspoon baking soda
1 teaspoon cinnamon
¼ teaspoon allspice
¼ teaspoon ginger
¼ teaspoon nutmeg
¼ teaspoon cloves
¼ cup (41 g) raisins
¼ cup (27 g) chopped pecans

Frosting
8 ounces (227 g) vegan cream cheese (e.g., Tofutti, Daiya)
½ cup (96 g) palm sugar (see Notes)
½ teaspoon vanilla extract
3 tablespoons cocoa powder
Plant-based milk, as needed

Optional garnishes
Chopped pecans, orange peels, and/or dark chocolate shavings

1. Preheat the oven to 350°F (180°C).
2. In a mixing bowl, combine the canola oil, vanilla, plant-based milk, honey, flaxseeds, and chia seeds and beat with an electric mixer or whisk vigorously for 2 minutes, until very smooth and fluffy.
3. Stir in the carrots.

4. In another bowl, blend the flour, baking powder, baking soda, cinnamon, allspice, ginger, nutmeg, and cloves. Add to the wet ingredients, a small amount at a time, stirring only to combine. Fold in the raisins and pecans.

5. Place 12 cupcake papers in a muffin pan and fill each with batter about three-quarters full.

6. Bake the cupcakes for 30 to 35 minutes, until golden brown and a toothpick inserted in the center comes out clean. Remove from the oven and let cool for a few minutes. Remove the cupcakes from the pan and cool fully.

7. Meanwhile, beat the vegan cream cheese, palm sugar, vanilla, and cocoa powder with an electric mixer or whisk until very smooth and fluffy. Add plant-based milk, 1 teaspoon at a time, if needed to create the desired texture.

8. Frost the cooled muffins and garnish as desired with chopped pecans, orange peels, and dark chocolate shavings.

notes: Skip the frosting for a healthier dessert or to serve as a muffin.

Palm sugar (also called coconut sugar or coconut palm sugar) is growing in availability and has a taste reminiscent of caramel. If you can't find it, substitute brown sugar in this recipe.

variations: Substitute chopped dates for the raisins, and walnuts, hazelnuts, or macadamia nuts for the pecans. To make this gluten-free, substitute a gluten-free flour blend (such as Bob's Red Mill or King Arthur Flour) for the white whole wheat flour, and ensure all other ingredients are gluten-free.

> **PER SERVING:** 278 calories, 5 g protein, 40 g carbohydrate, 13 g fat, 2 g saturated fat, 4 g fiber, 17 g sugar, 258 mg sodium
>
> **STAR NUTRIENTS:** thiamin (12% DV), vitamin A (55% DV), calcium (10% DV), copper (12% DV), iron (10% DV), magnesium (14% DV), manganese (60% DV), phosphorus (18% DV), selenium (22% DV)

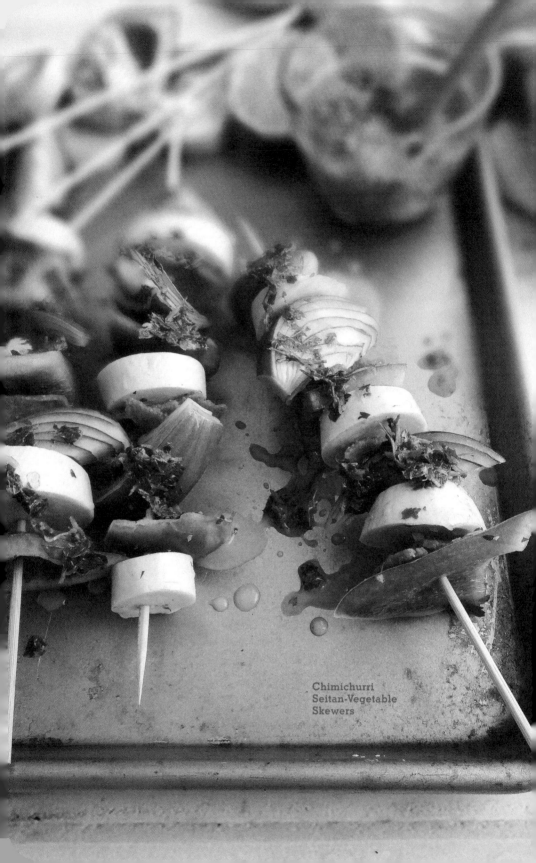

Chimichurri
Seitan-Vegetable
Skewers

Create a new plant-powered goal.

Chimichurri Seitan-Vegetable Skewers
Oven-Roasted Root Vegetables with Caraway
Savory Grain and Nut Loaf with Mushroom Sauce

Here you are, at the end of your plant-powered journey. I hope that you have found a new love and appreciation for plants, in all of their colorful, flavorful, textured, and nuanced glory. I hope that you have found recipes that have become new favorites, which will reappear on your table week after week. I hope that you've left a few smears on the recipes in this book and dog-eared your favorite pages as you took these plant-powered habits to heart. I hope that your children, parents, and friends have been pleasantly surprised to find that plant-based eating can be delicious. And I hope that you have learned a new trick or two about how to make optimal health sustainable for your whole lifetime.

And now I'd like to ask you to take a quiet step back and ask yourself what this experience has meant to you. Was it easy to introduce more whole plant foods into your diet? Does this eating style make you feel better? Do you have a better understanding of the foods that surround you? What's the next step for you?

Perhaps you'd like to continue on your plant-powered journey by further reducing your intake of animal foods—meat, poultry, fish, dairy, eggs—and increasing your fully plant-powered meals during the week. Or maybe you're ready to take on a pescatarian lifestyle, in which you say no to meat and poultry but maximize the benefits of eating fish a couple of times per week. That's fine, too. If you're ready to give vegetarianism a shot, and you'd like to do it the whole-foods, plant-powered way, instead of the processed, junk-foods way—that's super. And if you're really ready to take the plunge, and take on an entirely vegan lifestyle, relying only on plant foods to sustain you, that's wonderful. I'd like to give you a pat on the back as you make your way along your own plant-based path for life. More plant-power to you!

chimichurri seitan-vegetable skewers

ACTIVE PREPARATION TIME: 14 minutes • TOTAL PREPARATION TIME: 37 minutes
(not including marinating time)

Expand your plant-powered horizons by taking lessons from cultures around the globe. Chimichurri is an herbal, tangy Argentinean sauce traditionally used on grilled meats, but it shines on veggies and seitan, too. Savory, "meaty" seitan—essentially wheat protein—has its own culinary roots that date back to seventh-century China. Just thread chunks of summer squash, onions, bell pepper, and seitan onto skewers and grill (or oven-roast) them for a show-stopping entrée that's as delicious as it is attractive at your next party or backyard barbecue.

MAKES 4 SERVINGS
(1 skewer each)

2 medium garlic cloves
1 cup (60 g) packed cilantro leaves
½ cup (30 g) packed parsley leaves
Juice of 2 medium lemons
Juice of 2 medium limes
1½ tablespoons extra virgin olive oil
1 tablespoon agave nectar
1 8-ounce (227 g) container plain seitan, sliced (see Notes)
1 medium onion, sliced into wedges
1 small summer squash (e.g., crookneck or zucchini), thickly sliced
1 medium bell pepper, thickly sliced

1. Combine the garlic, cilantro, parsley, lemon and lime juices, olive oil, and agave in a food processor or blender. Process just until herbs are finely chopped (but not completely liquefied).

2. Prepare 4 skewers on metal or wooden skewers, alternating slices of seitan, onions, squash, and pepper. (Soak the skewers first, if using wooden.)

3. Place the skewers in a large, shallow dish. Pour the marinade over skewers and chill for 1 hour.

4. Heat the grill and cook the skewers for 8 to 10 minutes on each side, until the vegetables are crisp-tender. Brush the marinade over the skewers while grilling.

notes: You may also roast the skewers in the oven for 35 to 40 minutes (15 to 20 minutes on each side) in a 400°F (205°C) oven, brushing with the marinade a few times while cooking.

Seitan is a wheat-gluten meat substitute that is available in many supermarkets and natural food stores in the refrigerated section.

variations: Substitute mushrooms or eggplant for the summer squash. To make this gluten-free, substitute extra firm tofu (pressed, for best results—see page 000) for the seitan.

PER SERVING: 189 calories, 17 g protein, 22 g carbohdyrate, 7 g fat, 1 g saturated fat, 6 g fiber, 9 g sugar, 293 mg sodium
STAR NUTRIENTS: folate (10% DV), vitamin A (22% DV), vitamin B6 (13% DV), vitamin C (263% DV), vitamin K (218% DV), calcium (15% DV), copper (12% DV), iron (10% DV), magnesium, (13% DV), manganese (34% DV), phosphorus (13% DV), potassium (11% DV), selenium (12% DV)

oven-roasted root vegetables
with caraway

ACTIVE PREPARATION TIME: **16 minutes** • TOTAL PREPARATION TIME: **1 hour 26 minutes**

Pledge to fill your plate with even more vegetables. It's not hard—even when the cool weather arrives—when you focus on seasonal produce. Before potatoes gained attention in the Western world, root vegetables such as turnips, parsnips, and rutabagas were staples. Rich in fiber, un-refined carbs, and a host of important nutrients, these humble vegetables flourished in cooler climes and could last for months tucked away in a root cellar. No wonder they were such an important staple for hardwork-ing folks across Europe. In fact, roasted root vegetables are still an English tradition on Sundays. My simple recipe, flavored with aniselike caraway seeds, calls upon a variety of root vegetables. Make it your own Sunday roast tradition, paired with Savory Grain and Nut Loaf with Mushroom Sauce (page 340).

MAKES 8 SERVINGS
(¾ cup each)

1 medium rutabaga, peeled and diced
1 medium turnip, diced
1 medium parsnip, peeled and sliced
1 medium russet potato, peeled and diced
1 medium carrot, sliced
1½ tablespoons extra virgin olive oil
⅓ cup (79 ml) apple juice
1 teaspoon apple cider vinegar
2 medium garlic cloves, minced
1 teaspoon caraway seeds
½ teaspoon low-sodium herbal seasoning blend (see page 345)
¼ teaspoon freshly ground black pepper

1. Preheat the oven to 350°F (180°C).
2. Combine the vegetables in a 9 by 13-inch baking dish.
3. In a small dish, whisk together the olive oil, apple juice, vinegar, garlic, caraway seeds, herbal seasoning, and black pepper. Pour over the veg-etables and toss together.
4. Bake, uncovered, for about 1 hour 10 minutes, until the vegetables are tender and golden brown. Stir once or twice during the baking time.

variations: Substitute 1 small sweet potato for the russet potato; swap out the other vegetables according to what looks good at the market or the choices in your CSA box.

PER SERVING: 106 calories, 2 g protein, 19 g carbohydrate, 3 g fat, .5 g saturated fat, 4 g fiber, 8 g sugar, 48 mg sodium
STAR NUTRIENTS: folate (10% DV), vitamin A (23% DV), vitamin B6 (12% DV), vitamin C (55% DV), potassium (16% DV)

---

savory grain and nut loaf
with mushroom sauce

ACTIVE PREPARATION TIME: **35 minutes** • TOTAL PREPARATION TIME: **1 hour 20 minutes**

*Don't be afraid to try new things along your plant-powered journey—
even if they're a blast from the past. I grew up in a semi-vegetarian home
during the seventies, and my mom was a wizard at creating a rotation
of nut and cereal loaves for dinner. These loaves were all the rage back
then, and I think they're ready for the resurgence that other retro culinary trends are currently enjoying. The simple idea of combining whole
grains, legumes, nuts, vegetables, and herbs into a savory, baked, meat-
free loaf is brilliant. This home-cooked star of the dinner plate can be accompanied with roasted seasonal vegetables (see page 338) or steamed
greens.*

MAKES 8 SERVINGS
(2 slices each)

⅓ cup (64 g) dried small lentils
⅓ cup (63 g) uncooked quick-cooking brown rice
¼ cup (50 g) uncooked millet
¼ cup (48 g) uncooked amaranth
2¼ cups (474 ml) water
1 reduced sodium vegetable broth bouillon cube
1 tablespoon extra virgin olive oil
1 medium onion, finely diced
2 medium garlic cloves, minced
1 medium celery stalk, finely chopped
1 medium carrot, shredded
1 cup finely chopped mushrooms
1 medium green bell pepper, finely diced
½ cup (58 g) finely chopped walnuts
¼ cup (30 g) chopped fresh parsley, or 1 tablespoon dried
2 teaspoons poultry seasoning (see Notes)
Nonstick cooking spray
½ cup (78 g) uncooked old-fashioned oats
½ cup (54 g) whole grain bread crumbs (see Note on page 95)
1 tablespoon vegan Worcestershire sauce (see Notes on page 297)
1 tablespoon reduced sodium soy sauce
¼ cup (66 g) tomato paste
¼ teaspoon black pepper

Mushroom Sauce
1 teaspoon extra virgin olive oil
½ cup (35 g) diced mushrooms
1 medium garlic clove, minced

2 cups (474 ml) unsweetened plain plant-based milk
3 tablespoons all-purpose flour
1 tablespoon reduced sodium soy sauce
Pinch of freshly ground black pepper

Garnish
2 tablespoons chopped fresh parsley

1. Combine the lentils, brown rice, millet, amaranth, water, and bouillon cube in a small pot, cover, and cook for 25 minutes over medium heat, stirring occasionally. When tender but not mushy, drain any remaining water and transfer the mixture to a large mixing bowl.

2. Meanwhile, heat the olive oil in a large skillet or saucepan. Add the onion and sauté for 6 minutes, stirring occasionally.

3. Add the garlic, celery, carrot, mushrooms, bell pepper, walnuts, parsley, and poultry seasoning. Sauté for 8 minutes, stirring occasionally.

4. Preheat the oven to 350°F (180°C). Spray an 8 by 12-inch baking dish with nonstick cooking spray (see Notes).

5. Transfer the sautéed vegetables to the mixing bowl with the lentil mixture. Add the oats, bread crumbs, Worcestershire sauce, soy sauce, tomato paste, and black pepper. Stir well to combine.

6. Pour the mixture into the baking pan, cover with foil, and bake for 45 minutes. Remove the foil and bake for an additional 20 to 25 minutes, until golden brown on top and tender.

7. While the loaf is baking, prepare the mushroom sauce. Heat the olive oil in a saucepan over medium heat. Add the mushrooms and garlic and sauté for 3 minutes. In a small dish, whip together the plant-based milk, flour, soy sauce, and black pepper until smooth with no lumps. Pour the milk mixture into the saucepan and cook, stirring frequently, for about 8 minutes, until bubbly and thick.

8. To serve, slice the loaf in half lengthwise to create two rows, and then into 8 slices in each row for a total of 16 slices. With a spatula, carefully serve 2 slices of loaf onto a dinner plate. Ladle the mushroom sauce (about 4½ tablespoons per serving) over the slices and garnish with 1 teaspoon of freshly chopped parsley.

notes: Poultry seasoning, which is available at many supermarkets, is a vegetarian herb-spice blend that typically includes dried parsley, sage, rosemary, marjoram, black pepper, and onion powder.

You may use two 9 by 5-inch loaf pans instead of an 8 by 12-inch pan.

recipe continues

variations: You may substitute pecans, hazelnuts, or sunflower seeds for the walnuts. To make this gluten-free, use gluten-free broth, oats, bread crumbs, Worcestershire sauce, and soy sauce, and substitute 1½ tablespoons corn starch for the flour.

PER SERVING: 265 calories, 11 g protein, 35 g carbohydrate, 10 g fat, 1 g saturated fat, 7 g fiber, 5 g sugar, 363 mg sodium

STAR NUTRIENTS: folate (24% DV), niacin (18% DV), riboflavin (25% DV), thiamin (25% DV), vitamin A (32% DV), vitamin B6 (20% DV), vitamin C (81% DV), vitamin K (106% DV), calcium (13% DV), copper (19% DV), iron (18% DV), magnesium (19% DV), manganese (54% DV), potassium (17% DV), selenium (14% DV), zinc (10% DV)

Ingredients Notes

APPLESAUCE OR PEAR SAUCE

To make your own, combine 4 ripe medium apples or pears (peeled, cored, and chopped), ¼ cup water, juice of 1 small lemon, and ½ teaspoon cinnamon (if desired) in a pot. Cook, covered, over medium-low heat for about 30 minutes, until tender, then use a blender, food processor, or immersion blender, to process to your desired texture.

CANOLA OIL, EXPELLER PRESSED

To make expeller-pressed canola oil, the oil is obtained from the plant through mechanical processes, rather than through chemical processes, such as the use of solvents. Some chemical solvents may become environmental contaminants, which is why I recommend that you use expeller-pressed oils.

COCONUT MILK

When I call for "coconut milk beverage," I mean the kind that comes in a carton.

"Coconut milk" or "light coconut milk," on the other hand, is the kind that comes canned, often in the Asian section of the supermarket. The latter should always be mixed well before being measured, because it separates in the can.

PLANT-BASED MAYONNAISE

I recommend you use highly processed ingredients only sparingly, but vegan mayonnaise can provide a nice creaminess to items such as dressings. You can find vegan mayonnaise (e.g., Veganaise) in many stores, but you can also make a more natural substitute yourself with the following recipe.

MAKES ⅔ CUP

½ cup unsweetened plain soy milk
1 tablespoon lemon juice
1 teaspoon Dijon mustard
¼ cup (59 ml) extra virgin olive oil
Pinch of sea salt (optional)
Pinch of white pepper (optional)

1. Combine the soy milk, lemon juice, and Dijon mustard in a tall narrow cup. Using an immersion blender for best results, whip the ingredients. Slowly add the olive oil, 1 tablespoon at a time, while whipping for about 4 minutes, until the mixture is foamy and thickened.
2. Pour the mixture into a container and refrigerate. It will thicken as it chills. Before using, season with a pinch of sea salt or white pepper, if desired.

PLANT-BASED SOUR CREAM

While vegan sour creams are available in supermarkets, you can also make up your own with my easy recipe.

MAKES ABOUT ¾ CUP

½ cup (113 g) silken firm tofu
1 tablespoon extra virgin olive oil
Juice of 1½ lemons
1 teaspoon white vinegar
Pinch of sea salt (optional)

1. Combine the tofu, olive oil, lemon juice, and vinegar in a blender or the work (may use immersion blender or traditional blender). Process until very smooth. Add a pinch of salt, if desired.
2. Chill until serving time; it will thicken slightly as it chills.

SEASONINGS

I use many herbal seasoning blends in this book. Here are some tips and instructions for making your own.

Cajun Seasoning: Cajun seasoning can give just the right kick to dishes but, like taco seasoning, can be high in sodium. Create your own by blending 2½ teaspoons paprika, 2 teaspoons garlic powder, 1½ teaspoons onion powder, 1½ teaspoons oregano, 1½ teaspoons thyme, 1 teaspoon black pepper, 1 teaspoon cayenne pepper, and ½ teaspoon crushed red pepper. Mix well and store in an airtight container.

Garam Masala: Garam masala is a traditional seasoning blend used in Indian cuisine. You can find it in many gourmet food stores or Indian food markets, or you can make your own by combining 1 tablespoon ground cumin with 1½ teaspoons each of ground coriander, cardamom, turmeric, and black pepper; and ½ teaspoon each of ground cloves, ginger, cinnamon, mustard, and nutmeg. Mix well and store in an airtight container.

Herbes de Provence: This traditional seasoning blend from the South of France can be purchased at many gourmet shops, but you can also make it yourself by combining equal parts dried savory, thyme, rosemary, basil, marjoram, oregano, whole fennel seeds, and lavender flowers. Mix well and store in an airtight container.

Low-Sodium Herbal Seasoning Blend: Many brands of special herbal seasoning blends are available, such as Mrs. Dash, Spike, and Bragg. They come in a variety of flavors, such as spicy or garlic and herb. I like to use an all-purpose blend to add a neutral flavor base in recipes, then add more of a particular spice to accent the recipe.

Low-Sodium Taco Seasoning: Taco seasoning blends can be delicious—and high in salt. So make your own low-sodium version by combining 1½ teaspoons paprika, 2 teaspoons chili powder, ½ teaspoon cumin, ½ teaspoon oregano, ¼ teaspoon black pepper, ⅛ teaspoon cayenne pepper, ⅛ teaspoon crushed red pepper, 1 teaspoon onion powder, and 1 teaspoon garlic powder. Mix well and store in an airtight container.

Za'atar: This is a traditional Middle Eastern spice used to add extra flavor to many dishes. To make your own in a food processor or spice grinder, grind together 1 tablespoon thyme, 1 tablespoon marjoram, 1 tablespoon oregano, 1½ teaspoons sesame seeds, and 2 tablespoons sumac. Store in an airtight container.

REDUCED SODIUM VEGETABLE BROTH

For every 1 cup of vegetable broth called for in this book, you can use 1 cup of reduced sodium canned or packaged vegetable broth (or stock); 1 teaspoon of reduced sodium vegetable broth base plus 1 cup of water; or half of a reduced sodium vegetable bouillon cube plus 1 cup of water.

Alternatively, make your own vegetable broth with the following recipe:

MAKES 7 CUPS

1 tablespoon extra virgin olive oil
1 large onion, chopped
3 medium carrots, chopped
2 celery stalks, leaves included, chopped
1 bell pepper, chopped
3 green onions, white and green parts, chopped
4 garlic cloves
8 cups (1,896 ml) water
½ ounce dried mushrooms
10 whole peppercorns
2 cups (48 g) assorted fresh herbs (parsley, sage, oregano, thyme, marjoram, basil, savory)
2 bay leaves
2 tablespoons reduced sodium soy sauce
Pinch of sea salt (optional)

1. Heat the olive oil in a large pot and add the onion, carrots, celery, bell pepper, green onions, and garlic. Sauté for 10 minutes.
2. Add the water, mushrooms, peppercorns, herbs, bay leaves, and soy sauce. Stir well, cover, reduce the heat to medium, and simmer for 1½ hours.
3. Taste and add a pinch of sea salt, if desired. Strain the soup and use the vegetables as a side dish or refrigerate for later use.
4. Use the broth immediately or refrigerate for up to one week. Leftovers can also be frozen.

Further Reading

For additional resources on plant-based eating, please refer to some of my favorites.

Loma Linda University (www.lluedu.com), my alma mater, is performing incredible research on the power of plant-based eating in their Adventist Health Studies. These landmark studies are documenting that this eating styles is good for health, as well as for the environment.

Meatless Monday (www.meatlessmonday.com) is a great starting place for plant-powered inspiration. Going meatless one day a week is a simple, achievable goal we can all benefit from.

Oldways Vegetarian Network (www.oldwayspt.org) provides science-based information on eating a balanced, plant-based diet centered on delicious, traditional foods. I'm proud to be a nutrition advisor in this organization.

The Vegetarian Resource Group (www.vrg.org) is your go-to spot for everything you need to know about eating a healthful, plant-based diet.

Seasonal Recipe Guide

Recipe Name	Spring	Summer	Fall	Winter
Apple and Fennel Salad with Arugula (page 192)			✓	✓
Applesauce Raisin Snack Cake (page 224)	✓	✓	✓+	✓+
Artisanal Nut and Seed Spread (page 213)	✓	✓	✓	✓
Arugula Salad Pizza (page 10)	✓	✓+	✓+	
Baked Potato and Leek Soup (page 274)	✓	✓	✓+	✓+
Banana-Coconut Brown Rice Pudding (page 238)	✓	✓	✓+	✓+
Banana-Walnut-Flax Bread (page 280)	✓	✓	✓+	✓+
Bell Pepper Rye Pilaf (page 54)		✓	✓	
Black Bean and Corn Chili (page 236)	✓	✓	✓+	✓+
Black Bean Brownies with Walnuts (page 317)	✓	✓	✓	✓
Black Bean, Cilantro, and Avocado Quesadillas (page 184)	✓	✓	✓+	
Blueberry Oatmeal Waffles (page 190)	✓	✓	✓	✓
Bombay Carrot, Beet, and Bulgur Salad (page 142)	✓	✓	✓	✓
Borscht with Beets and Beet Greens (page 232)	✓	✓	✓	✓
Broccoli-Mushroom Gratin (page 294)	✓	✓	✓	✓
Buckwheat Tabbouleh (page 164)	✓	✓	✓	
Butternut Squash and Caramelized Onion Salad (page 330)		✓	✓	✓
Cajun Rattlesnake Beans with Corn (page 256)	✓	✓	✓+	✓+
California Tofu Scramble (page 244)		✓	✓	
Caribbean Calypso Beans (page 24)		✓	✓	
Carrot Spice Cupcakes with Chocolate "Cream Cheese" Frosting (page 332)	✓	✓	✓	✓
Cashew Cheese with Popped Seeds (page 328)	✓	✓	✓	✓
Chana Dal Stew (page 193)	✓	✓	✓+	✓+
Chickpea Stew with Kale and Za'atar (page 12)	✓	✓	✓	✓
Chile Hot Chocolate (page 316)	✓	✓	✓	✓+
Chimichurri Seitan-Vegetable Skewers (page 336)		✓	✓	
Creamed Spring Peas and Potatoes (page 216)	✓	✓		
Creamy Peanut Butter Pie (page 222)	✓	✓	✓	✓
Crispy Ginger-Amaranth Cookies (page 150)	✓	✓	✓	✓
Crunchy Farro-Hemp Breakfast Bowl with Fresh Berries (page 282)	✓	✓		
Curried Tofu Papaya Wraps (page 144)	✓	✓	✓	
Easy Peanut Soba Noodles with Seitan (page 50)	✓	✓	✓	✓
Edamame Hummus (page 148)	✓	✓	✓	✓

Recipe Name	Spring	Summer	Fall	Winter
Endive Salad with Peas, Pea Shoots, and Creamy Lemon Dressing (page 60)	✓	✓		
Ethiopian Yam and Lentil Stew (page 91)		✓	✓+	✓+
Farro and White Bean Veggie Burgers (page 36)	✓	✓	✓	✓
Fettuccine with Romesco Sauce (page 4)	✓	✓	✓	✓
Fig Oat Bars (page 114)	✓	✓	✓	✓
Flower and Pomegranate Tea (page 307)	✓+	✓+	✓	✓
Forest Berry Salad with Juniper Vinaigrette (page 264)	✓	✓		
French Lentil Salad with Cherry Tomatoes (page 26)		✓	✓	
Fresh Guacamole with Tomatoes and Serrano Chiles (page 205)	✓	✓	✓	
Fruit and Almond Breakfast Shake (page 288)	✓	✓		✓
Ginger-Cardamom Baked Acorn Squash (page 217)			✓	✓
Green Bean Casserole with Caramelized Onions (page 16)		✓	✓	
Grits Smothered with Mustard Greens (page 246)		✓	✓	✓
Haricots Verts, Tomato, and Almond Salad (page 32)		✓	✓	
Harvest Wild Rice Salad with Persimmons and Baby Spinach (page 170)			✓	✓
Hot Spiced Wine with Raisins and Almonds (page 325)	✓	✓	✓+	✓+
Jicama-Chayote Slaw (page 46)		✓	✓	
Kiwi Herb Salad with Pistachios and Orange Dressing (page 302)	✓		✓	✓
Korean Kimchi Hot Pot (page 310)	✓	✓	✓	✓
Lemon-Lavender Cooler (page 305)	✓	✓	✓	
Lentils with Wild Mushrooms and Broccoli Rabe (page 230)	✓	✓	✓	
Mediterranean Eggplant and Artichoke Lasagna (page 94)		✓	✓	
Miso-Braised Collard Greens with Cashews (page 43)		✓	✓	✓
Moroccan Vegetable Tagine with Couscous (page 180)	✓	✓	✓	✓
Muhammara (page 177)	✓	✓	✓	✓
Orange Millet Scones (page 71)	✓	✓		✓
Oven-Roasted Root Vegetables with Caraway (page 338)		✓	✓+	✓+
Pantescan Potato Salad (page 125)	✓	✓	✓	
Peach and Cranberry Crumble (page 107)		✓	✓	
Peanut Butter and Banana Quinoa Breakfast Bowl (page 137)	✓	✓	✓	✓

NOTE: ✓ indicates that the produce used in a recipe is well suited to the season. ✓+ indicates the recipe is especially well suited. Seasons vary depending on your geographic location. This list is based on information from the USDA and US farmers market guides and is relevant to most residents of the United States.

Recipe Name	Spring	Summer	Fall	Winter
Pear Buckwheat Pancakes (page 138)	✓	✓	✓	✓
Pecan-Cherry-Chia Nutrition Bars (page 206)	✓	✓	✓	✓
Persian Couscous with Apricots and Pistachios (page 69)	✓	✓	✓	✓
Pesto Trapanese with Whole Grain Penne (page 120)	✓	✓	✓	
Pigeon Peas with Pumpkin and Sofrito (page 200)		✓	✓	✓
Pineapple and Mango with Coconut (page 58)	✓	✓		
Pinto Bean and Tofu Breakfast Rancheros (page 136)	✓	✓	✓	
Polenta with Puttanesca Sauce (page 84)	✓	✓	✓	✓
Portobello Mushroom and Spinach Pie (page 296)	✓	✓	✓	✓
Pumpkin Spice Muffins with Pumpkin Seeds (page 130)	✓	✓	✓+	✓+
Red Bean and Okra Jambalaya (page 18)		✓	✓	
Red Lentil Soup with Root Vegetables and Sage (page 178)		✓	✓+	✓+
Roasted Cauliflower with Freshly Ground Spices (page 126)	✓	✓	✓	✓
Roasted Chickpeas with Spices (page 30)	✓	✓	✓	✓
Roasted Lemon-Dill Asparagus and Tofu (page 102)	✓	✓		
Roasted Lemon-Sage Brussels Sprouts with Hazelnuts (page 62)		✓	✓	✓
Rosemary and Olive Cassoulet (Bean Stew) (page 86)	✓	✓	✓	✓
Ruby Winter Quinoa Salad (page 67)				✓
Rustic White Bean and Sun-Dried Tomato Toasts (page 186)	✓	✓	✓	
Savory Grain and Nut Loaf with Mushroom Sauce (page 340)	✓	✓	✓	✓
Savory Shiitake and White Bean Bake (page 292)	✓	✓	✓	✓
Scandinavian Apple-Cardamom Oatmeal (page 212)			✓	✓
Seeded Whole Wheat Biscuits (page 210)	✓	✓	✓	✓
Sesame Udon Salad with Snow Peas (page 20)	✓	✓		
Shanghai Stir-Fry with Forbidden Rice (page 2)	✓	✓	✓	✓
Sicilian-Style Eye of the Goat Beans (page 96)	✓	✓	✓	✓
Smoky Chili with Sweet Potatoes (page 198)		✓	✓	✓
Spaghetti Squash with Pomodoro Sauce and Pine Nuts (page 44)	✓	✓	✓	✓
Spicy Black-Eyed Pea Salad (page 162)	✓	✓	✓	
Spring Vegetable Salad with Green Goddess Dressing (page 300)	✓+	✓	✓	
Sprouted Lentil Granola with Apricots (page 322)	✓	✓	✓	✓
Steel-Cut Oats Risotto with Asparagus (page 38)	✓	✓		

Recipe Name	Spring	Summer	Fall	Winter
Stir-Fried Barley with Sea Vegetables and Peanuts (page 132)	✓	✓	✓	✓
Stone Fruit Trifle (page 218)		✓		
Strawberry Soy Lassi (page 276)	✓	✓		
Strawberry-Macadamia Shortcake (page 100)	✓	✓		
Summer Succotash with Heirloom Tomatoes (page 258)		✓+	✓	
Sun-Dried Tomato and Olive Chickpea Focaccia (page 154)	✓	✓	✓	
Swedish Pea Soup (page 118)	✓	✓	✓+	✓+
Sweet Potato and Pecan Maple Pie (page 226)			✓	✓
Sweet Potato Gnocchi with Pistachio-Orange Pesto (page 74)			✓	✓
Teff Porridge with Dates, Figs, and Pistachios (page 166)	✓	✓	✓	✓
Tempeh Noodle Skillet with Bok Choy (page 252)		✓	✓	✓
Thai Lettuce Wraps (page 240)	✓	✓	✓	
Toasted Chickpea Sea-Salad Sandwiches (page 312)	✓	✓	✓	
Tofu Cobb Salad (page 82)	✓	✓	✓	
Tofu Mushroom Tacos (page 8)	✓	✓	✓	
Tofu Ratatouille (page 250)	✓	✓	✓	
Tomato Barley Soup (page 263)	✓	✓	✓	✓
Tortilla Soup (page 112)	✓	✓	✓	
Tropical Green Smoothie (page 289)	✓+	✓+	✓	✓
Tropical Red Cabbage and Spelt Salad (page 77)	✓	✓	✓	✓
Truffled Mashed Gold Potatoes and Celery Root (page 270)	✓	✓	✓	✓
Tuscan Fusilli with Swiss Chard and Fava Beans (page 172)	✓	✓	✓	✓
Tuscan Kale Salad with Nectarines and Brazil Nuts (page 269)		✓		
Vegetable Ribbon Salad with Lime Vinaigrette (page 158)	✓	✓		
Watermelon-Basil Ice (page 106)		✓		
Whipped Hazelnut Iced Coffee (page 306)	✓	✓	✓	✓
Yellow Squash Stuffed with Saffron Rye Berries (page 156)	✓	✓	✓	
Zucchini Verde Sprouted Rice (page 320)	✓	✓	✓	
Zucchini-Orzo Soup (page 52)	✓	✓	✓+	

NOTE: ✓ indicates that the produce used in a recipe is well suited to the season. ✓+ indicates the recipe is especially well suited. Seasons vary depending on your geographic location. This list is based on information from the USDA and US farmers market guides and is relevant to most residents of the United States.

Acknowledgments

I would like to express my appreciation to so many people who have inspired this book along its journey. From the start, my publisher, Matthew Lore, and editor, Molly Cavanaugh, from The Experiment, who really *get* plant-powered eating, had an amazing vision for my book. We dreamed of a book that would help people attain simple, easy habits that would form the core of plant-based eating for optimal health. And we wanted this book to be filled with gorgeous, globally inspired, delicious food, which was brought to life through the artistry of Heather Poire, a photographer who also truly understands the beauty of whole plant foods. My agent, Linda Konner, was there every step of the way, guiding this dream book to fruition. And my friends, who cheered me on through the *Plant-Powered Diet*, never missed a beat as I moved on to *Plant-Powered for Life*. My family, Peter, Christian, and Nicholas, spent a year of their lives giving me the thumbs-up or thumbs-down on hundreds of plant-powered concoctions at our dinner table. They were right when they told me to ditch the vegan mocha cheesecake and that my jambalaya recipe was amazing. My husband took *The Plant-Powered Diet* to heart, and as a result got off statins. And my teenage sons don't complain too badly when I make them eat fruits, vegetables, and whole grains at every meal (they'll thank me for it someday!). Thanks also to all of the farmers who have worked tirelessly over the generations, saving the seeds from their very best plants and cultivating them year after year, so that I might enjoy something as precious as a ripe Brandywine tomato on a hot August day. Most of all, this book is for the thousands of people who have found such joy and vibrant health in plant-powered living. The club of plant-powered eaters is growing strong; it *is* the future, and I'm happy to be a part of it.

Index

Page numbers in *italics* refer to photos.

About the Author

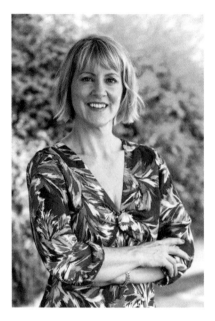

SHARON PALMER, RDN, is a registered dietitian, editor of the award-winning health newsletter *Environmental Nutrition*, author of *The Plant-Powered Diet*, and a nationally recognized nutrition expert who has personally impacted thousands of people's lives through her writing and clinical work. She lives outside of Los Angeles with her husband and two sons.